DR CLAIRE WEEKES

M.B.E., M.B., DSc., F.R.A.C.P.

ESSENTIAL HELP

for your

NERVES

Recover from nervous fatigue
and overcome stress and fear

Thorsons

Thorsons
An Imprint of HarperCollins*Publishers*
77–85 Fulham Palace Road,
Hammersmith, London W6 8JB

The website address is: www.thorsonselement.com

More Help for Your Nerves
First published in Great Britain by
by Angus and Robertson (UK) in 1984
First published by Thorsons 1995
This revised edition 2000

Peace from Nervous Suffering
First published in Great Britain by
Angus and Robertson (UK) in 1972
First published by Thorsons 1995
This edition 2000

18

© Claire Weekes Publications 2000

Hazel Claire Weekes asserts the moral right to
be identified as the author of this work

A catalogue record for this book is
available from the British Library

ISBN-13 978-0-7225-4013-8
ISBN-10 0-7225-4013-2

Printed and bound in Great Britain by
Clays Ltd, St Ives plc

Essential Help for your Nerves

Contents

Preface

Our family is very proud of the legacy left by our aunt, Dr Claire Weekes. Dr Weekes' aim was to give nervously ill patients control back over their lives. She provided information, self-help techniques and comfort, both in person and through her lectures, writings and tapes. Her empathetic guidance lives on in this combined edition of her books *More Help for your Nerves* and *Peace from Nervous Suffering*.

Even now, after her death in 1990, I still receive letters from patients she has helped. One woman in America wrote recently that, after recovering from nervous illness by reading Dr Weekes' books, she became a doctor and has since been in practice for twenty years. People often write to say how much her books have helped them and are still helping them.

Dr Weekes was a trailblazer in the field of self-help and her books are as relevant now as they were when she wrote them. Her books were originally written over thirty years ago and have never been out of print.

Dr Weekes dedicated her life to helping hundreds of thousands of people worldwide. She has left a legacy of life-giving hope and practical strategies for achieving complete wellbeing.

Frances J Maclaren
Canberra
September 1999

BOOK 1

MORE HELP

for your

NERVES

Contents

To my sister, Dulcie Maclaren, for her courage and love; to my friends, Joyce Skene Keating, J.P., Irene Appleton and Steven Reich, for their great effort and devotion to the work and to the memory of Elizabeth Coleman, who always put obligation before inclination and love and loyalty before all else.

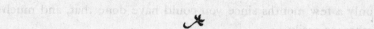

CHAPTER 1

Nervous Fatigue

- ℱ Muscular Fatigue
- ℱ Emotional Fatigue
- ℱ Mental Fatigue
- ℱ Fatigue of the Spirit

Understanding nervous fatigue is the key to understanding the baffling experiences that make recovery from nervous illness so elusive – within grasp one minute, gone the next. Understanding is the forerunner of cure.

Nervous fatigue can show itself as one, or more, of four fatigues: muscular, emotional, mental and a kind of fatigue of the spirit, and these often develop in this order.

That sounds straightforward enough, yet few people recognize these fatigues in themselves because their development has been so gradual, so insidious. And yet, this development follows a consistent pattern which is the basis of so much nervous suffering.

Indeed, recognizing fatigue as an important part of their illness can bring such relief to so many, their subsequent recovery can be straightforward and simple. I said simple. I did not say easy.

At this moment, while you read this, you may be bewildered by what is happening to you. Perhaps the task of facing today, tomorrow, seems too much for your exhausted body to attempt, too much for your tired mind to think about. And yet it may be only a few months since you could have done that, and much more, so easily.

You may have reached the stage where you feel you would rather close your eyes and never open them again than have to open them tomorrow. All this may be so unlike your old self – indeed may seem to be a reversal of that former self – that your bewilderment may be extreme.

When I explain to some bewildered, nervously ill people that their suffering is based on nervous fatigue, they are at first dubious that such strange, disturbing symptoms as theirs, such utter exhaustion, could have such an apparently simple cause. However, when convinced, being nervously fatigued seems less frightening than the 'mental' illness they were beginning to suspect was theirs. Their picture of mental illness has so many dark, mysterious places.

The difference between nervous fatigue and nervous illness must be explained. A person can suffer from one, or all, of the four fatigues – muscular, emotional, mental and 'spiritual' – and still, in my opinion, not be nervously ill. It is only when he becomes *afraid of the effects* of fatigue and allows this fear to interfere with his life, that I say he has passed from being nervously fatigued to being nervously ill.

Of course there are many different kinds of nervous illness. In this and in my books, *Self Help for Your Nerves, Peace from Nervous Suffering* and *Simple, Effective Treatment of Agoraphobia*, I am concerned mainly with the simplest and most common kind: the anxiety state.

Anxiety is closely related to fear. The difference between them is one of timing as well as of intensity. For instance, in an acute emergency – such as facing an immediate danger – we would say we were afraid, whereas when contemplating a threatening future event we would say we were anxious rather than afraid.

The term 'anxious' comes from the Latin *anxius* meaning being upset about some future uncertain happening. So, literally, being in an anxiety *state* should mean being in a condition of prolonged anxiety. However, in practice, a person in an anxiety state is both anxious and afraid and is very often particularly afraid of his nervous symptoms.

I say 'particularly afraid of his symptoms' because there are two main types of anxiety state. In the first, the original stress has passed and is no longer responsible for the illness. The sufferer is now concerned with fear of the symptoms this original stress brought. He is afraid of the state he is in, caught in a maze of fear from which he cannot free himself. So his continuing anxiety state is based on fear of symptoms.

In the second type, the sufferer is more concerned with some problem, or problems, that may have caused his illness and is not cured until this, or these, are resolved. Peace of mind about his problems is usually essential for his cure.

In my practice the vast majority of people were of the first type. They were afraid of their nervous symptoms and often also of the strange experiences stress brought, and in this book I am mainly concerned with them. However, my teaching about understanding nervous fatigue also helps people with a specific problem, or problems (even those with a subconscious cause of illness) – it gives them an understanding of their symptoms and experiences, which at least clears some bewilderment and so opens the way to recovery.

As mentioned earlier, as long as a nervously fatigued person is not unduly anxious about, or afraid of, his condition, he is *not*, in my opinion, in an anxiety state, not nervously ill.

Regardless of whether a person is nervously ill or merely nervously fatigued, he will benefit from understanding the four fatigues. Even those people who have never suffered from nervous fatigue can be protected from it by understanding it.

So let me guide you, as I have guided so many, to an understanding of nervous fatigue and to recovery from any existing nervous illness.

MUSCULAR FATIGUE

The First Fatigue

Ordinary muscular fatigue is easy to recognize. It may come after strenuous exercise, when it's good to relax – especially in a hot bath – and enjoy the aching muscles that speak so satisfyingly of achievement. However, the muscular fatigue that comes with nervous fatigue is not enjoyable. It comes, not from the extra use of muscles, but from their abuse – from subjecting them to too constant and too severe tension.

Resting muscles are usually in a condition called tone, which is a state balanced between relaxation and contraction; in this way, they are kept ready for use. Tone is maintained by reflex nervous arcs; for example, were you to sit and cross your legs at the knees and tap the crossing leg, just below the kneecap, it would automatically jerk. You couldn't stop this because the action is a reflex; what is more, your leg could jerk that way all day without becoming tired. Reflex action is not tiring. However, *prolonged tension in muscles upsets tone* – the balance between relaxation and contraction – *and also allows the chemicals of fatigue to accumulate. So, aching begins.*

This is perhaps the main reason why nervously ill people so often complain of aching legs, aching back, aching neck and, less frequently, of aching arms.

The ache from tension is persistent, and should its victim have to stand, perhaps for only a few minutes, he will look around for support, preferably somewhere to sit, even lie, to relieve those heavy, aching, dragging legs. And yet there is nothing organically wrong with those legs: they are only fatigued through tension.

A feeling of weakness can also follow tension. Bend your right leg at the knee and fiercely tense it. Hold it that way for 30 seconds and then release it. Even after such a short spell of tension, it may feel shaky. The weakness of those shaky legs of nervous fatigue has such simple explanation.

BLURRED VISION

Muscular fatigue can also affect the delicate muscles that accommodate the lens of the eye, so that vision may be blurred, especially on looking quickly from a near to a far object and vice versa. Also, objects in bright sunshine may appear as if in shadow. Although perhaps frightening, these upsets are temporary and unimportant: however, the sufferer with no knowledge of fatigue may think he is going blind and fear further attacks.

ALL-OVER HEADACHES

Tension in neck and scalp muscles can cause headache which may extend from above the eyes, over the top of the head, to the base of the skull and into the neck. There may also be very tender spots over the temples, at the base of the skull and down the sides of the trapezius – the stout muscle that helps support the head and anchor it to the body.

In addition, the head may feel so heavy, the scalp muscles so sore, that resting comfortably on the pillow at night may be difficult without a painkiller. For permanent cure, tension itself must be eased. However, knowing that tension is the cause of the pain (not brain tumour!) relieves some anxiety and hence some tension.

Much has been written today about removing tension, stress, by practising relaxing exercises. For nervously fatigued and nervously ill people, I recommend such exercise, at first directed by a competent teacher. If this is not practical I suggest discussion with their doctor.

We can be too anxious about always being relaxed and so may become tenser than usual. I advise relaxing at a set time, once or twice daily, and then worrying no more about it for the rest of the day. Such a daily routine can be built into our subconscious.

Relaxing through subconscious programming is more successful than becoming tense through constantly trying to remember to relax!

How we sit, stand and lie can be revealing. Trying to support the head in an uncomfortable position – for example, reading in bed or in a chair with an uncomfortable back – tenses head and neck muscles.

Having one's eyes on another job before finishing the one in hand is another guarantee of tension. A whirlwind can propel a toothbrush to finish its job when its owner spots dust on the shelf above the basin. Here again, the subconscious can be harnessed to help. Short, daily, routine practices at moving (cleaning teeth!) slowly will be enough to calm the whirlwind.

Although I mention treatment here, I reserve discussion of further treatment of the four nervous fatigues until the chapter on Recovery.

EMOTIONAL FATIGUE

The Second Fatigue

If during stress our body always remained calm, we would feel no emotional fatigue and there would be many fewer sufferers of nervous illness. However our body doesn't work that way. When nerves are subjected to stress, especially to strong emotions such as fear, for a long time, they can be aroused to record emotion with increasing intensity and often with unusual swiftness. They become trigger-happy and fire off at the slightest provocation. I call this aroused state *sensitization*. Sensitization of nerves is a most important part of nervous fatigue and consequently of nervous illness – of the anxiety state in particular to which, in my opinion, it is so often an important contributing cause.

When nerves are severely sensitized, emotion – especially fear – can seem to strike with physical force. The sufferer, rarely recognizing this as sensitization, becomes bewildered and afraid of it and so puts himself into a fear-adrenalin-fear cycle. *This is the crucial point where so many people pass from being simply sensitized to becoming nervously ill.*

To understand the fear-adrenalin-fear cycle we should understand how our nervous system works. Although I describe this in earlier books, it is necessary to include a brief description here.

FEAR-ADRENALIN-FEAR CYCLE

Our nervous system consists of two divisions: voluntary and involuntary. By means of voluntary nerves we move our muscles more or less as we wish. The voluntary nerves are under our direct command – hence their name, voluntary.

The involuntary nerves, with help from our glands, control the functioning of our organs: heart, lungs, bowels and so on.

Unlike the voluntary nerves they, with a few exceptions, are not under our direct control – hence their name, involuntary. However, they respond to, and register, our moods; for example, when afraid, our cheeks may blanch, our heart race and our blood pressure rise. We don't consciously do this and – what is so important in understanding nervous illness – we have no power to stop these reactions other than to change our mood. Research workers are experimenting today (for example, with relaxation, meditation) to try to control involuntary reaction; so far their results still depend on calming mood.

The involuntary (sometimes called autonomic) nerves themselves consist of two divisions: sympathetic and parasympathetic. In a peaceful body these two hold each other in check. However, when under stress (for example, when we become angry, afraid, excited) one division dominates the other. In most people the sympathetic dominates the parasympathetic. These are the people whose heart races, blood pressure rises and so on. This is called the fight-or-flight response.

Sympathetic nerves are activated by hormones. A hormone, as defined by *Collins Concise English Dictionary*, is a substance formed in some organ of the body and carried to another organ or tissue, where it has a specific effect. Several hormones are involved in sympathetic reaction to stress, but for the sake of simplicity I will speak only of adrenalin, the best known and perhaps the prime mover of all the hormones released by sympathetic nerves.

Occasionally, under stress, parasympathetic nerves dominate: pulse rate decreases, blood pressure falls. However, more usually the reaction is sympathetic, not parasympathetic, and when I speak of the fear-adrenalin-fear cycle I mean sympathetic reaction.

In my earlier books I called the sympathetic nerves, 'adrenalin-releasing nerves', and will do so here, because they are certainly not 'sympathetic', as we understand that word.

Among his many different symptoms, a sensitized person under stress, as well as feeling his heart beating unusually quickly, may feel it 'thump', 'miss' beats; he may have attacks of palpitation, feel his body vibrating with what he may describe as an electrical buzz; feel tremor, muscle jerks, muscle weakness, tingling in his limbs, churning stomach, light-headedness and so on, and above all, a spasm of fear may be felt as a flash of panic.

These symptoms can be so bewildering and upsetting that the sufferer may become more afraid of them than of the cause of his original stress.

Surely it can be understood how, by adding the extra stress of fear to his original stress, the sufferer stimulates the release of more and more adrenalin (and other stress hormones) and so further intensifies the symptoms he dreads, *which are themselves the symptoms of stress*.

This is the fear-adrenalin-fear cycle into which a sensitized person can easily be trapped and so placed on the way to nervous fatigue; perhaps nervous illness.

It is easy to add fear-of-fear when an original spasm of fear is felt as a scorching flash. Naturally the sufferer recoils from the flash and as he recoils, adds a second flash. I call these two fears first- and second-fear. Indeed, a sensitized person may be more concerned with his physical feeling of fear (usually panic) than with the original danger that brought it, and because that old bogy sensitization prolongs the first flash, the two fears may feel like one. This is why a sufferer fails to recognize the two separate fears and so, fails to see how he prolongs his illness by adding the second fear. He resensitizes himself with every spasm of second-fear. For him there is no greater enemy than his lack of understanding.

A nervously ill person may become so afraid of his symptoms that he may avoid places where he thinks stress will bring them. Therefore, he may become afraid to leave the protection of his home. This condition, called agoraphobia, is becoming more widely recognized today. In my opinion, it is no more than a *particular stage* in an anxiety state. I discuss this in detail in my book, *Simple, Effective Treatment of Agoraphobia.*

It is important to understand that a person in an anxiety state (whether agoraphobic or not) may have continuous underlying sensitization because he constantly resensitizes himself with anxiety and fear. SENSITIZATION IN A PERSON WITH NO FEAR OF IT, WOULD HEAL ITSELF.

As mentioned earlier, I stress the importance of sensitization because it is the forerunner of emotional fatigue and therefore possibly also of nervous illness. The sequence is: stress (either sudden or gradual), then sensitization, then bewilderment and fear. These are followed eventually by emotional fatigue and the added complications this brings – all possibly appearing finally as nervous illness.

Sensitization is the prime cause of emotional fatigue because, when severe, it exaggerates *all* emotions and so gradually depletes the sufferer's store of emotional energy. Having all emotions exaggerated is bewildering indeed and is one of the main reasons why a sensitized person sometimes thinks he must be going mad. For example, a slightly sad sight can seem tragic; a gloomy sight, overwhelmingly eerie; impatience can be felt as agitation; noise amplified until it seems intolerable; even a moment of joy can be felt hysterically. A sensitized person, feeling emotion as intensely as this, must inevitably become emotionally fatigued, feel 'drained'.

A nervously fatigued woman anxiously watched her old mother slump dejectedly as she walked up the garden path to a taxi waiting to take her to her one-roomed apartment and loneliness. Normally the daughter could have comforted herself with the thought that she would often visit her mother, would take her out, get her to join the Senior Citizens Club, perhaps get her interested in a hobby; but now in her sensitized anguish she could not convince herself of any of this. For her, there seemed only heartbreaking anxiety, and she wondered how long she could survive it.

Another nervously fatigued woman, while sight-seeing in England, visited some Roman Baths. These could seem a bit gruesome to anyone, but to her they were so eerie should could hardly restrain herself from running outside. She was bewildered by her strong reaction. I explained that sensitization had exaggerated her feelings and that her agitated revulsion was only an intensified, sensitized version of the normal queasy feeling that anyone would get in the same situation.

GUILT

Most of us have some guilt tucked away that we have learnt to live with without letting it upset us too much – but not so the sensitized person. Guilt shouts so loudly at him he feels he will never be reconciled to it. He sees no light at the end of that tunnel. Also, even if he struggles successfully with one guilt, sensitization will soon present him with another. He has only to think of some guilt, perhaps up until now long forgotten, to immediately feel that frightening *whoosh*.

Some therapists say that a patient who comes with a list of guilty worries is 'that kind of person' – always looking for something to worry or feel guilty about. He may be, but more likely he is sensitized. Unfortunately, instead of an explanation of sensitization, tranquillisers are too often the only remedy prescribed.

Also, some therapists make too much of guilt simply because the patient does; so while the sufferer may take only one or two small guilts to his therapist, he may leave with a heavy bundle.

The impulse to confess guilt is strong while emotional and fatigued; the urge to be relieved of that heavy load on the chest is so insistent. However, a sufferer should beware of yielding to such an urge while sensitized. Confessing guilt can sometimes complicate, not comfort. How essential it is to understand sensitization. I discuss coping with guilt in Chapter 3.

THUNDER IN THE STREET

Sensitization can also exaggerate noise. Heavy vehicles can sound like thunder in the street and sitting through a noisy movie can feel like torture. The person, who does not understand that noise is temporarily amplified by sensitized auditory nerves, is naturally bewildered and this is increased by the strength of the force that grips and incites him to 'rush away from it all'.

LOVE INTENSIFIED

More bewildering still (as if he hasn't had enough already!), even pleasant experiences can be exaggerated; for example, the intensity of the love felt at no more than the sight of a loved one's hand can move the sensitized person to tears.

JOY FELT HYSTERICALLY

And, as already mentioned, a rare moment of joy can be felt hysterically. A nervously ill man described how, on one occasion when standing beside a piano while a friend played the accompaniment to a rollicking song, he joined in the singing.

When they finished, his friend turned and said, 'Don't tell me you're depressed and ill! You sang that better than any of us. You seemed deliriously happy!' The man explained to me, 'Doctor, if they only knew! While I was singing I felt more manic than happy. In fact, delirious was the right word. That was how I felt. If only I could stay just a little bit happy and not the way I am – way up one minute and down the next. They haven't a clue, doctor!'

THE SHOCK OF WAKING

Also a sensitized body can react to the slightest shock. Even the mild shock of waking from sleep can make a heart race. This may be accompanied by such a strong feeling of foreboding the sufferer may need to keep reassuring himself that nothing terrible has happened, or is about to happen.

Such a person, fearing anxiety so intensely, may become so susceptible to it that the mere hint of its approach can grip 'the pit of his stomach' with a gnawing ache – and how he longs for a comforting word to ease that ache. Sensitization can be a real stomach-gripper!

Also, while he is so responsive to anxious thought, the slightest hazard his imagination may conjure up seems overwhelming; for example, if he tosses at night and cannot sleep, the sensitized person easily imagines he will never be able to sleep properly again. And what a response he gets from his sensitized body!

Because of such flashing response to any anxious thought, he may feel powerless to make decisions, be embarrassingly suggestible and so become gradually bereft of confidence. At this stage he may feel as if his personality has disintegrated, as if both he and the world are unreal.

We describe some people with exaggerated reactions (not necessarily nervously fatigued or nervously ill) as unbalanced, and a sensitized person certainly feels this way. He may feel this imbalance so acutely that he begins to think he is some sort of weakling. One man said desperately, 'I am the exact opposite to what I used to be, to what I really am. What is happening?' He did not understand that this feeling of imbalance was temporary and was no more than his body's sensitized expression of ordinary, normal emotion. Small wonder that one so buffeted by emotion is incredulous when told that his suffering is no more than sensitized nerves exaggerating normal reaction and that when freed from the effects of tension, sensitization can heal itself. This is why understanding sensitization and the part it plays in causing emotional fatigue is so important: UNDERSTANDING IN ITSELF RELEASES SOME TENSION.

The exhaustion following prolonged, exaggerated emotional reaction (especially if accompanied by upsetting physical nervous symptoms: quickly beating heart, 'missed' heartbeats, churning stomach and so on) is especially bewildering because (1) it can seem so incapacitatingly severe and yet be so little related to physical effort and so little relieved by resting and (2) is so difficult to describe and so rarely understood by those who have never felt it, including the family and even doctor.

One nervously ill woman said, 'I feel as if my whole body is a "nothing", doctor! I haven't the strength to pull it together and yet my husband keeps saying, "For God's sake, pull yourself together Jess! How can you be so tired, when you've done nothing all day?"'

We can survive long periods of stress providing that our glands – principally pituitary and adrenal – can continue to supply essential hormones. The body adapts to stress. However, if adaptation fails (glands become depleted) we pass to the stage of exhaustion. This is why emotional exhaustion – based on glandular depletion – is not appreciably related to physical effort nor appreciably helped by rest, but is almost miraculously helped by release from emotional suffering and so from stress.

Apathy and depression warn of approaching depletion. First comes apathy. As I say in my book, *Self Help for Your Nerves*, even to comb his hair can become such an effort that the sufferer begins to look unkempt and no longer cares.

With further depletion, apathy becomes depression. The depression of nervous illness is almost invariably caused by emotional depletion.

The symptoms and experiences I have been describing may sound frightening. However, they are less frightening when one understands the simple pattern of their development and that recovery lies in reversing that pattern, as I show later. There is no particular bogy; no compelling outside force. There is only a body's natural reaction to stress – and the body will react just as naturally by healing itself when stress is removed. And much stress is removed simply by understanding.

MENTAL FATIGUE

The Third Fatigue

The sensitized, fatigued person is naturally concerned about himself, 'how he feels', so his anxious thoughts often (sometimes constantly) turn inward. Much anxious introspection brings mental fatigue, just as concentrated study can bring brain-fag in a student. Arthur Rubinstein, speaking at the Juilliard School of Music, advised pupils to practise no more than three or four hours a day; any longer, he said, was wasted time because the mind could not absorb it.

When the mind is fresh, thoughts can flit lightly from subject to subject. In a severely mentally fatigued person, thoughts come haltingly and sometimes so slowly that thinking is an effort, almost as if each thought has to be selected and placed individually in the sentence. Speech may therefore be hesitant, even sometimes stuttering.

The sufferer may also become confused and find concentrating and remembering difficult. Forgetting immediate events can be so persistent the sufferer may suspect he is going prematurely senile.

Talking can be such a strain for a mentally tired person that if he sees a neighbour approaching he will cross the street rather than talk to him. He may sometimes begin a sentence and feel too tired to finish it.

Before he was so mentally tired, he could spend hours on the weekend sitting in the sun, lazily dipping into the newspapers, scarcely thinking at all as time slipped by, but now he watches time consciously, almost every second of it. And how those seconds drag; an hour can seem like eternity to a mentally fatigued person.

Normally we rest our mind during the moments when we look and listen without concentrating too intensely; unimportant thoughts flit so lightly from subject to subject we are hardly aware of them: the funny design on the new ironing-board cover, the shine on the leaves of the copper beech tree. However, when mentally fatigued thoughts do not flit, they seem to stick. This is one reason why a mentally tired person gnaws at a worry, feeling unable to release it, especially if the worry holds fear.

When thoughts 'stick' and are accompanied by fear, the way is prepared for the development of obsessions, phobias. So many obsessions and phobias *begin in this simple way*.

An obsession is a thought that preoccupies a mind to an abnormal degree and this is exactly what can happen to a sensitized person suffering from mental fatigue, when a repeated 'sticky' thought that frightens comes with such force that it seems to propel its victim almost physically. Surely it is understandable how obsession can be born at this point? Understanding this is extremely important because with understanding, obsession loses its mystery and so, some of its power to frighten.

A fairly common obsession is doubt about loving one's spouse. A nervously ill woman said that although she knew she really loved her husband, the thought that she didn't kept recurring so frequently and with such force, she was beginning to think it was true. Of course it was her sensitized response to this fear and its repetition in her tired mind that was convincing her. When sensitization and mental fatigue come together, throwing off frightening thoughts can seem impossible.

This woman found that her inability to disregard her upsetting thoughts, although in her heart she knew them to be false, was one more proof that she was going mad. How many nervously fatigued, or nervously ill, people have thought this! And of course, the more frightened she felt, the more sensitized she became and the more overpowering and persistent were her thoughts.

She admitted that the thought about not loving her husband was most convincing and stuck most tenaciously when she was tired. She also said there were moments when she could see this thought for what it really was: no more than a silly thought in a very tired mind. At such times the idea seemed so absurd, she could smile at it. I call these flashes of normal thinking, *glimpsing*. I discuss curing obsession by glimpsing in a later chapter.

A phobia is an irrational, persistent fear. This can develop very simply in a sensitized person. While mental fatigue makes the development more likely, sensitization alone can be enough. A sensitized person, while waiting in a queue, instead of feeling normal exasperation, can feel agitated panic and from then on may avoid standing in any queue, so developing a queue phobia. In this simple way many phobias arise. Understandably simple, isn't it?

A mentally fatigued person may say his mind feels enveloped in a blanket, feels dull, heavy, thick. This may be aggravated by blurred vision and perhaps a tendency to stagger slightly (accompanying muscular fatigue). Some say they feel as if a good hard crack on the head would clear it.

In mental fatigue an attack of muzzy head may last from a few hours, to days. As one woman described it, 'I seem to have a wall in my head that my thoughts knock against. It's very hard to concentrate; before, I always had a very clear head and good insight. But this muzzy head! When it clears I can think very well, but when it descends, I'm finished!

'I had a guilty experience about which I worried so much, I couldn't get worry off my mind. My psychiatrist told me that I was punishing myself and put me on medication. This helped, but this 'thing' came back again. I would have a clear head for half an hour and in that time I could talk, even laugh, and then all of a sudden, I would remember the guilt, start crying inwardly and the muzzy head would descend.'

Not recognizing her muzziness as a combination of brain-fag and tension, she became alarmed by it, and so added to her problem stress, more tension, more brooding and therefore, more brain-fag.

While imprisoned by his blanket of mental fatigue, a sufferer, because of slowed thinking and muzzy head, may become aware of a pressing consciousness of self – especially of his actions, his thoughts. This inward-thinking, as I call it, may persist after most of the other symptoms of nervous illness have gone; indeed, it is sometimes the last symptom with which he has to contend.

He rarely recognizes it as that old bogy, mental fatigue, still at work, binding his mind in the tracks it has been following for the previous months or years.

Exasperation at being caught in this trap brings more inward-thinking, more stress, more tension – a frightening cycle – and the harder he tries to escape from it, the more bound within it he feels.

This cycle of fatigue and sensitization working together *is following simple, natural laws that can be reversed*. Inward-thinking can be cured, as I show later.

SUDDEN GLARE SHOCKS!

A mentally fatigued person, especially when used to the shade and shelter of indoors, can feel sudden shock on opening the front door and facing the light. In my book, *Self Help for Your Nerves*, I described a mentally fatigued, nervously ill man who was obliged to pass through a dark tunnel before emerging on to a sunlit beach packed with people and gay umbrellas. He was so shocked by the sudden brightness, he felt unreal, like a sleep-walker. The shock arrested his thoughts and gave him insight into the greyness of the world he had been living in – a world of constant anxious introspection – and he *recognized this greyness as no more than persistent mental fatigue*.

The experience helped him recover. For the first time he understood the meaning of mental fatigue, and became aware of how absorbingly bound he had been in his own anxious thoughts. He could see now that his trouble was not so much the gravity of his problems as the fatigued state he was in. This came as a revelation because for weeks he had been desperately gnawing at those problems thinking that they were insoluble. Understanding helped release him.

FATIGUE OF THE SPIRIT

The Fourth Fatigue

Finally, there is fatigue of the spirit. When a nervously fatigued person is so depleted that every action, perhaps every thought, is an effort, he begins to wonder if the struggle is worth it. Some say they feel as if they have been suddenly precipitated into old age; that they haven't the strength to face another day, let alone weeks, months. The will to survive falters, especially if the sufferer has been trying to recover by fighting his way out of fatigue. The best way to increase fatigue is to try to fight it, as I will show in the next chapters.

First, the fatigued spirit must somehow find fresh hope and courage. The merest glimmer is enough to begin with. It may have to be, because even that can seem too much for an exhausted spirit to resurrect. However, recovery can build on such a slender foundation, so slender, that at the slightest puff of discouragement, it may seem to collapse.

And yet, if there is understanding and a plan for recovery instead of a hopeless no-man's land, hope and courage do grow again, as bravely as the green shoots grow on the burnt-out tree-stumps in a forest ravaged by fire.

I have seen so many people take those first shaky steps to recovery holding desperately on to such slender hope and courage, sustained by the understanding I have been privileged to give them.

Although those first steps may seem weak and faltering, they hold the same indomitable strength that has carried us all through millions of years of our evolutionary struggle.

We all have this strength, this power, within us, and it will work miracles if we trust it to help us learn to walk and live with fear, so that we can eventually walk and live without fear.

So, on, brave spirit.

CHAPTER 2

❊

Recovery

❊ Facing
❊ Accepting
❊ Floating
❊ Letting time pass

It may be difficult for a sufferer from nervous fatigue to appreciate the difference between his fatigue and nervous illness. Some – particularly executives struggling to hold down an important and stressful job, indeed anyone trying to do a day's work that seems beyond their ability to cope – may suspect that, if not already suffering from nervous illness, they are at least threatened by it. So they have two struggles, one with their fatigue and another with their fear of it becoming illness. This struggle is particularly poignant because in their exhausted state their fear of nervous illness can open the door to it.

Understanding his symptoms and experiences will at least relieve the nervously fatigued person of bewilderment. Also, with understanding he is less likely to become afraid of 'the state he is in' and although perhaps tottering with fatigue, can keep himself free from actual nervous illness.

However, if fear, through ignorance, takes control, the fatigued person often flounders in despair, almost blindly reaching for help. At this time the right guidance is crucial. Many years of experience in helping hundreds of nervously fatigued and nervously ill people have proved that the guidance I now offer, if followed, will bring peace.

I teach recovery from nervous fatigue and nervous illness by using four simple concepts: facing, accepting, floating and letting time pass. Although I have discussed these in previous books, many readers have continued to ask questions about them; so I will discuss them here in further detail.

It becomes confusing to talk about nervously fatigued and nervously ill people and at the same time try to differentiate between them. So, henceforth, I will speak to the nervously ill, although stressing that much of the advice given applies equally to the nervously fatigued.

FACING

Facing means acknowledging that cure must come from inside you – with guidance and help from outside, of course – but fundamentally by your effort, and this means by your facing the things you fear. RECOVERY LIES IN THE PLACES AND EXPERIENCES FEARED.

Facing also means not shying away from nervous symptoms *for fear of making them worse*. Shying away is running away, not facing.

Recently I met a striking example of not facing in a Canadian who panicked when away from home and who was consequently afraid to travel any distance from home, either alone or accompanied.

His therapist encouraged him to go out as far as he could without panicking. If he panicked (and he surely would), he was told to return home and repeat the journey later, still going only as far as he could with comfort. The therapist's aim was for the patient to become so used to that particular journey that he could eventually make it without panic.

This man managed so well, he decided to spend his holiday in the United States. He spent two weeks in Las Vegas and did not panic. He returned home in triumph.

The next day he went down to his bank; the same bank he had visited so often when ill. He stood on the old familiar spot in the queue, and as he handed his bank-book to the same teller – the one with the thick rimmed glasses – memory smote and he panicked. *And this time it was a smasher,* because with the return of panic came despair. He had managed so well before going away, and yet all he need do now was simply stand in the queue in his own bank for panic to sweep once more. No wonder he despaired and thought, 'What can I do *now*!' He was desolate.

He had found peace only by getting-used-to. He had never faced panic, had never learnt how to cope with it fully. He had been taught to avoid it, to try to quieten it, never how to pass through it until *it no longer mattered.*

It is true that some people feel they have been helped by avoiding, but *they are vulnerable to returns of panic.* At the return of even a slight spasm, their brave little flag can crumple.

I stress again, and again, that in place of an inner voice that says hopefully, 'Perhaps it won't happen here', there must be a supporting voice that says, 'It doesn't matter if it *does* happen here. It just doesn't matter any more. You can cope with it!' The voice that says, 'Perhaps it won't ...?' is the sword of Damocles, waiting.

While I never teach the 'getting-used-to' technique to people afraid of travelling away from home (called agoraphobic), it has its place in treating people with specific phobias, such as fear of cats, thunderstorms, heights and so on. Behaviourists build a programme of graduated exposure to a feared object that can not only relieve, but often cure this kind of phobia.

Also, it is possible to get so used to some nervous symptoms that they no longer matter. Then without the stress of mattering, they may, of course, calm, even disappear.

I also said facing means accepting that cure must come from within oneself and not from some permanent outside crutch. This means recognizing that the way to recovery can be difficult. A journalist wrote in a magazine that she had been agoraphobic for years, but could now go anywhere providing she took a special tablet three times a day. 'Now,' she wrote, 'I have only to come off the tablets and I am cured!' She had only to stop taking tranquillizers! In other words, while still lame, she had only to throw away her crutches and walk.

Whether she could do this would depend on her luck the first time she tried to go out without her tablets. If she was confident, and stayed confident, all could be well, but she needed only a slight shiver of doubt for panic to strike and all could be lost. This applies to the return of all the symptoms of nervous illness, when tranquillized away. Tranquillization merely postpones the time when symptoms must be faced to be cured. There is a place for tranquillization but it should be chosen with discretion. I talk more about this later.

The permanent cure of nervous illness based on fear of symptoms and experiences – as so much nervous illness is – begins by facing fear itself, especially at the peak of its intensity. THE RIGHT WAY.

While facing fear blindly is brave, it is too often futile and exhausting. For recovery, the sufferer must be shown how to face fear *by accepting, floating, and letting time pass*.

ACCEPTING

After becoming prepared to face, the next step is acceptance, and as acceptance is the key to recovery, we should be sure of its meaning. Acceptance means letting the body loosen as much as possible and then going toward, not withdrawing from, the feared symptoms, the feared experiences. It means 'letting go', 'going with', bending like the willow before the wind – rolling with the punches!

When one goes forward this way into panic (into *any* of the feared symptoms), the secretion of the hormones (principally adrenalin) producing the symptoms is reduced. Even if only slightly, *it is reduced*. On the other hand, tense withdrawal encourages further secretion and so, more sensitization, and therefore, more intense symptoms.

While at first acceptance of physical symptoms, especially panic, may seem impossible, practising thinking about acceptance is always possible and this alone can release some tension (although perhaps only a microscopic amount to begin with), so that when 'it' comes to do its worst, the worst is tempered. If you stand taut and say bravely with clenched teeth, 'Come and do your worst! But get it over quickly!', you are only putting-up-with.

A patient will complain that he has accepted but that the dreaded symptoms are still there. 'I have accepted the churning in my stomach but I still have it! So what do I do now?' How could he have accepted, while he still complained about it?

The most frightening symptom is panic because, in a sensitized person, it can strike so fiercely and so quickly, merely thinking about it apprehensively can bring it on. The natural reaction is to recoil, to tense against it, to try to stop the flash coming; however, tension brings more sensitization and so, more panic. Acceptance is a definite physiological process that eventually soothes. I say eventually, because the soothing can rarely be felt immediately. Acceptance is the beginning. Established sensitization can rarely be soothed quickly, because it takes time for the new mood of acceptance to be felt as peace.

Although the symptoms of nervous illness are always the expression of mood, they are not always an expression of the present mood. When acceptance is first practised, the body may still be registering the tense, frightened mood of the preceding weeks, months, years and may continue to do this (but with progressively reduced intensity) even after the mood of acceptance is established.

This is why nervous illness can be so puzzling. A nervously ill person may begin to accept, but when the symptoms do not quickly disappear, he loses heart and becomes apprehensive once more, although trying to convince himself that he is still accepting.

I repeat, it takes time for a body to establish acceptance and for this to bring peace, just as it takes time for fear to be established as continuous tension and anxiety. This is why letting time pass, the last of my four concepts, is so important in treatment.

Understanding makes acceptance so much easier. It is unnecessarily difficult to accept erratic heartbeats if the victim believes that his heart is diseased. How much easier when he understands that the unevenness of those beats is no more than a temporary and unimportant upset in their nervous timing.

Adequate explanation is indeed a boon to the patient preparing to accept. However it is not always given. One woman said, 'I can't describe how I feel. I just feel funny. The doctors just look at me and give no explanation!' 'Feeling funny' can be an accurate description of how a nervously ill person does sometimes feel and describing his 'funny' symptoms can be difficult, because symptoms of fatigue and anxiety when working together can be vague, undefined, and vague symptoms can be just as upsetting as more definite ones.

If you feel like this, providing your doctor has examined you and said that your 'funny' symptoms are nervous, accept them and be comforted to know that funny feelings are common in nervous illness and never important. Blind acceptance can cure as well as acceptance based on knowledge; but when knowledge guides, acceptance is easier.

Some doctors, while knowing that 'funny' symptoms are 'nervous' do not understand their physiology and so cannot explain them. So, while 'funny' nervous feelings should be accepted without full explanation (if none is available), explanation of more definite symptoms (weakness, trembling, headache, palpitations, difficulty in swallowing and so on) should be sought. I explain these in detail in my first book, *Self Help for Your Nerves*.

Don't think I use the word acceptance lightly. I know what I am asking. It's not easy to accept the fire that consumes; not easy to work with the fire burning. It's not easy to accept and work with a body that feels as if it is vibrating, shaking; with stomach churning, limbs aching, heart pounding, sight blurred, head swimming ... I'm making it sound terrible, aren't I? It can be terrible and it is made worse if the mind, at the same time, feels as if it is drawn out into a frail thread that will snap with the slightest extra tension. I understand all this, but I still preach acceptance.

Recently a woman phoned to say that that morning had been especially rough for her. She'd come through by saying to herself, 'I'll be talking to Dr Weekes in a couple of hours. I'll have some peace then!' The thought of the peace to come sustained her. But living for such peaceful moments was not good enough; it meant that she would make little progress. There is no lasting peace in waiting for someone else to bring it. Such relief from suffering is only a respite.

I explained to this woman that peace lay within herself, and depended on her attitude when the symptoms were at their fiercest, and that that was the moment for her to practise the acceptance that would help her find lasting peace.

She thought for a while and then said, 'You mean I have to find the eye of the hurricane?' She had the message at last. Sailors say that at the centre of the hurricane there is a place of peace which they call the 'eye'. The storm swirls around but cannot reach it. To find it the ship must first go through the storm.

If that woman were to work as willingly as possible, accepting the symptoms (the hurricane) and *not add second-fear*, she would find the eye of the storm herself, and although the symptoms may at first seem as fierce as ever, there would be some peace and reassurance in knowing that she was on the right course at last, without having to wait for the doctor's soothing words.

Peace of mind built on earned confidence lies not in the absence of symptoms but in their midst, and it is only when one discovers this that the intensity of symptoms abates and there is peace. The process, of course, is gradual. The next day the woman reported that while feeling 'ghastly', she had sat at her work (she was an artist) and had painted for two hours. For the first time for months, she was able to lose herself in the work, while the hurricane raged within. For once the hurricane did not seem so important.

It takes courage to face the storm and let happen what will. That woman had been shrinking from the way she felt for 20 years and was still ill. Surely it was time she tried another

Essential Help for your Nerves

approach; tried to go into the storm, accepting it willingly – well, as willingly as she could manage at first.

Many are helped by understanding that the flash of panic is no more than an electric discharge; that while it may feel devastating, it is only an electrical discharge along sensory nerves. SO MANY PEOPLE ALLOW AN ELECTRIC FLASH TO SPOIL THEIR LIVES BY WITHDRAWING FROM IT IN FEAR.

As I have explained so often, fearful withdrawal produces the hormones that stoke the fire of panic. Facing and relaxing toward, with acceptance, help to dampen the flow and eventually stop it.

A sensitized, bewildered person, feeling his panic grow stronger as his sensitization increases, may imagine being flooded by an irresistible tidal wave of panic.

He should understand that there is a limit to the severity of even his panic. If he analyses his fiercest flash – the flash he thinks too fierce to bear – he will find that at its peak, *he is shudderingly withdrawing from it.*

WHENEVER HE FEARS PANIC HE CAN EVENTUALLY QUELL IT ONLY BY GOING FORWARD INTO IT, NEVER BY WITHDRAWING FROM IT.

A person sustained by this knowledge will one day be surprised by feeling panic sweep over him and yet FEEL ALOOF FROM IT, as if looking down on it. HE HAS LOST HIS FEAR OF PANIC. We talk about 'rising above a situation'; there is no better example.

When there is no longer fear of panic, it gradually subsides. Time becomes the healer. I stress again, and again, that cure lies in *losing* fear and that this is earned only by learning how to go through it the right way – with acceptance. With such understanding, it is possible to be cured immediately. I have seen this – but, of course, rarely.

Repeated panics can be exhausting. This is when I advise moderate and temporary tranquillization and an occasional rest, on sedation, to help the sufferer regain strength and refresh his spirit.

Tranquillization must always be planned so that the sufferer still earns his inner supporting voice born from having faced and accepted.

I talk so much about panic, because I am using it as an example from a hierarchy of nervous symptoms: palpitations, churning stomach, trembling hands and so on. When the sufferer learns to accept these without adding second-fear, they also gradually subside. They must, because they too are the symptoms of fear.

You may ask, 'But what if the nervously ill person is kept constantly stressed, perhaps frightened, by some problem – perhaps an upsetting domestic situation that is difficult to change? How can accepting the nervous symptoms help him? It can't solve the problem!'

It can't. However, people who develop nervous symptoms because of the stress brought by a problem, can also be further upset by the symptoms themselves; the iron-band headache, extreme fatigue, quickly beating heart, sweating hands and so on. Surely, understanding the nature of these symptoms helps lessen fear of them and so gives greater opportunity to concentrate on trying to solve any problem.

If you are reading this because you are nervously ill, I want you to practise acceptance now. Make yourself comfortable, take a deep breath, let it out slowly, let your tummy muscles sag, give way and try to feel a willingness to accept. Try to feel this in the pit of your stomach. Practise now.

Did you have a fleeting feeling of acceptance? If you did, you felt the birth of recovery. Continued acceptance will gradually finish the job.

It is necessary to understand the difference between true acceptance and putting-up-with. Putting-up-with (although calling for much bravery) means resistance. It means advancing and retreating at the same time. As I said earlier, it is an attitude of 'Hurry! Come quickly and get it over!' True acceptance means facing and relaxing, being prepared to go slowly with as little self-induced agitation as possible. It is submission.

I have used acceptance again and again in writing and recordings. You may think I place too much importance on it. How could I when it is the key to recovery?

I have said so often that peace lies on the other side of panic: now I shout it. By going through panic to the other side you earn the little voice that says, 'It doesn't matter any more if panic comes!' This is the only voice to listen to. It is your staff, and will always come to your help in setbacks, even if you find yourself almost helpless on the floor. As it lifts you up, you will feel again that the dreaded bogy no longer matters. As this realization strengthens, courage returns and you once more find the confidence to practice utter, utter acceptance – perhaps even more willingly.

Acceptance means throwing away the gun and letting the tiger come if he wants to. It sounds terrible, doesn't it? Incredible that cure can lie in such a dangerous procedure; but it does.

Just as facing and accepting are closely related, so are acceptance and floating. Indeed they are so close that sometimes distinguishing between them is difficult.

Let us now examine floating.

FLOATING

In the past, orthodox psychiatric treatment rarely recognized the importance of fear-of-fear and too often persisted with searching for childhood causes, which was neither necessary nor helpful.

One woman wrote, 'Not one psychiatrist, or psychologist, I visited would listen to the validity of the "fear-of-the-fear" and yet I am living proof of it. They were like stone and you can't reason with stone.'

So, disappointed and confused, perhaps made apathetic with heavy medication, nervously ill people often abandon treatment and, with little hope, sink further into their illness. Some try to treat themselves.

Unfortunately, self-treatment often fails because instinct too readily leads the sufferer in the wrong direction. He tries to *fight* his illness. HE SHOULD FLOAT, NOT FIGHT.

Many ask, 'What do you mean exactly by floating, doctor?' I can explain best by giving examples. A nervously sensitized person can become so supertensed with fear that he may stand immobilized, rigid, feeling unable to take another step forward, whether trying to walk along a street, enter a shop, or simply go from room to room at home. He rarely recognizes this 'paralysis' as supertension. Indeed, *his instinct is to tense himself still further and try to force his way forward.*

Forcing means more tension and therefore more rigidity. In his despair he may add panic to panic and when he does, his thoughts may seem to recede (they may actually seem to squeeze up into the back of his head) and become 'frozen' until further thought seems impossible. His 'brain goes numb'.

Agoraphobic people know and dread this moment of rigid 'paralysis' when trying to move away from home, and fear of it has helped to keep thousands housebound for years.

If the 'paralysed' sufferer, instead of forcing, were to let his body go as slack as possible (and actually feel as if it was sagging), then take a deep breath and exhale slowly while imagining himself *floating forward* without resistance – almost as if floating on a cloud or on water – he would release enough tension to loosen muscles and would be able to move forward, although maybe at first shakily, haltingly.

Another example of floating: a nervously ill person may wake in the morning feeling so tired he may shrink at the thought of the effort of getting out of bed, dressing, eating – indeed, of doing anything.

He may try to 'pull himself together' and this may seem so impossible that he sinks, defeated, back onto the bed. One woman said she felt like an ant looking at Everest.

Instead of seeing only grim effort ahead, she should think, 'Okay, I'll make the effort *as gently as I can*. "I'll go with it". I'll try to make no tense effort; I'll submit to it all, let it all happen. I'm not going to fight my way through any of it. I'll stop struggling and try to let my body float up out of it. I'll even float my clothes on.'

Can you appreciate the difference here between fighting and floating? Floating means no grim determination, no clenched teeth; as little 'pushing', forcing, as possible.

You may say, 'Floating is only relaxing!' It is certainly relaxing, but it is more than that; it is relaxing *with action*. One faces, relaxes and then floats on through.

Floating does not mean lying and gazing at the ceiling and thinking, 'I don't have to make any effort, I'll give up the struggle. I'll just lie here on the bed forever and do nothing!' That's relaxing all right! But it's not relaxing with action. And yet, *temporarily* 'doing nothing about it' can have a beneficial, refreshing effect – but only temporarily.

The sufferer practising letting his body float up from his fatigue has no need to search for a way to recovery. It is as if he steps aside from his body and lets it find its own way out of the maze. The body that so skilfully heals a physical wound without our direction can also heal sensitized nerves if given a chance and not hindered by inquisitive fingers picking at the scar. Float, don't pick.

Too often the same difficulties arise again and again in nervous illness and the repeated effort of fighting the same battle can make the sufferer feel too dispirited to go on searching for a way out. WHERE FIGHTING IS EXHAUSTING, FLOATING — BY REMOVING THE TENSION OF FORCING — MAKES REPEATED EFFORT LESS DAUNTING.

If, when learning to float, loosening a tense body may seem impossible, the supertensed person can at least *imagine* himself loosening. Even this works.

As I have already mentioned, people in an anxiety state can be grouped into those who have a special problem, or problems, causing illness and keeping them ill, and those whose only problem is finding a way to recovery from their distressing nervous state.

Those with the specific problem are not expected to float past it, although I have been quoted as having asked this of them. Expecting a bewildered, confused person to find his own answers to his problem is rarely good therapy. It can mean an unnecessarily long period of suffering because too often, through sensitization and fatigue, the sufferer switches too easily and too quickly from one point of view to another. Holding one point of view that brings some peace is essential for recovery. A good therapist helps his patient find such a viewpoint.

It is rare to meet a nervously ill person who can float past an agitating problem and worry no more about it. I did say in my first book, *Self Help for Your Nerves*, 'try to let all disturbing, obstructive thought float away, out of your head', but of course, success here depends on the magnitude of the troublesome thought. When I gave that advice previously, I referred to floating past one's own destructive suggestion. I did not mean the nervously ill should try to float past real problems.

This is one patient's experience of facing, accepting and floating: 'I feel I must write and tell you of the progress I have made this year. For 20 years, since my first attack of panic, I have been agoraphobic. During all these years, at the sight, or mere mention, of the word "bus", my stomach would turn over and the idea of getting on one – impossible!

'As you know, last year I got your cassette,* *Going On Holiday* (your records are worn thin with playing). As a result of constantly listening to the cassette, I decided to face a short cruise for myself and family.

'This year I booked a much longer cruise (a month!) to the Canary Islands. So, it was on with the cassette again. The first four days were not so good. The sea was rough and there was a strong wind. However, I had made up my mind to do everything I have been unable to do for so long. I went six times in the coach to the restaurant *alone*. I went up the mountains at Tenerife, 4000 feet, with a sheer drop on either side. I even crossed to the shore by launch.

'Only one evening was spoilt. When I entered the dining room that night. I had a terrible feeling of self-consciousness. I just couldn't swallow and it was my favourite meal, roast turkey! I did the only thing I could think of: I ate the soft vegetables and the desert and kept repeating to myself, "Loosen your body! Accept and float! Accept and float!" By the time we had reached the coffee I was floating fine.'

* For a full list of Dr Weekes' cassettes and recordings, and information on where to obtain them, see p. 425.

So now practise floating and while you do be prepared to obey the next section, and let time pass.

LETTING TIME PASS

Recovery, like all healing, must be given time. Understandably the nervously ill person is impatient with time and wants immediate appeasement; but impatience means tension and tension is the enemy of healing.

The sufferer removes a big obstacle to recovery when he understands that sensitization is a chemical process and needs time for chemical readjustment. A still sensitized body can be deceptively calm in a calm atmosphere but a body even only slightly sensitized cannot always maintain calmness when under renewed stress. So time, more time, must pass. Time itself is a healer. It's rather like the donkey and the carrot. The carrot (recovery) must be shifted just a little further forward during each setback but always remain within sight.

I am often asked how long recovery will take. So much depends on the degree of sensitization and the circumstances of recovery. There may be constant strain; for example, trying to recover while living with an upsetting domestic situation. Also it takes time to blunt memory's cutting edge. We can't anaesthetize memory. Indeed, when surprised by some gruelling memory, who can suppress an inner shudder? And yet, the person trying to recover from nervous illness seems to think he should. He wants the balm of constant peace.

It is difficult to understand that a body's sensitized reaction to memory is no more than the working of a natural law; difficult to understand that a setback is not always a setback in the sense that it sets *back*, but should be even expected and accepted *as part of recovery*. Its victim is much more likely to believe that some strange jinx is bugging him. His jinx is his lack of understanding. When so close to past upsetting experiences, and with a body still tuned to give a too quick, too intense, reaction to memory's prodding, it is natural to be too easily bluffed by memory into thinking he will never recover.

When memory first strikes it is as if the sufferer has learned nothing from past experience. The symptoms he'd learned to disregard suddenly begin to matter again – very much. And before he has time to study himself enough to think clearly, he feels sucked willy-nilly into the whirlpool of setback. However, if he had originally worked his way out of suffering the hard way – by having truly faced and lived with his symptoms while accepting them, having conquered adding second-fear (fear of symptoms, especially fear of panic) – then memory of his original recovery gradually awakens the little inner voice that says, 'You've come out of it before. You can do it now! You know that these symptoms do not really matter!' He hears this voice with thanksgiving and relief, because with it comes a special feeling, a realization that the symptoms really do *not* matter. He now *feels* this; doesn't just *think* it as he did at the beginning of setback. *He now feels it with relief.* Fear gradually goes; relaxation and peace come. He is on the way to true recovery. Recovery is built on *repeated* experiences of discovering that symptoms no longer matter.

When enough setbacks bring enough such experiences, the feeling of symptoms-no-longer-mattering comes more quickly, is more forceful, and the impact of memory's shock becomes weaker and weaker until it is but an echo of former suffering.

It is possibly because memory can shock by bringing back old symptoms so vividly, that some therapists speak pessimistically about complete recovery. Indeed they do not recognize that setback is one of the best teachers, and an almost essential halting place in recovery because it gives more time to relearn and practise. Not understanding this, they fail to prepare their patients optimistically for possible setback.

At some point in nervous illness the sufferer may be so ill he no longer cares what happens; however, as he begins to recover, caring returns and this may be complicated by his feeling that although much better, he cannot face the future demands and responsibilities of normal living. At such a time he is often accused of 'not wanting to get better'. Make no mistake, he wants to recover, but at the same time the prospect of coping with the demands of recovery may be so frightening while he is in his present state of only partial recovery, that he almost convinces himself that the criticism may be true – another bewilderment in nervous illness!

Enough time must pass to provide a protective layer of normal responses to help him gradually find his balance in normal living, to take normal reaction for granted.

As his body strengthens, his spirits rise, optimism and confidence return. The process may be so gradual he may be unaware of it. As I said in *Self Help for Your Nerves* 'It is this gradualness that makes all possible and only the passage of enough time can bring such gradualness.'

A Dutchman once said to Vera Brittain (an English author) that the postwar Dutch were suffering from a spiritual sickness which time and understanding alone would heal. He said that suffering could not be erased the moment the war ended and peace came; time was necessary for the Dutch to regain their balance, their ability to be on top of events, including their own lives. He added; 'Be patient with us. We have to grow into liberty.' And so must the nervously ill person grow into recovery. There is no electric switch, no overnight cure.

When the sufferer is beginning to recover, he is not only vulnerable to memory, but also is particularly vulnerable to the tricks any remaining fatigue may play. For example, distinguishing between normal fatigue and some remnant of nervous fatigue can baffle. The sufferer is apt to mistake any fatigue as nervous and jump to the upsetting conclusion that recovery is further away than he had thought. One woman, although much better, was so apprehensively suggestible, that when she made foolish mistakes playing bridge, she always blamed lingering illness and became worried. But she had made foolish mistakes at bridge before she was ill! Many nervously ill people expect recovery to bring a state of peace they never previously felt.

As already mentioned, for many people peace is often further delayed by their too fearful, and too tense, recoil from a binding awareness of self – the result of months, even years, of concentration on themselves and their illness. They delay their own recovery by trying to force forgetfulness. *Nothing can be forced in nervous illness.* The only way to lose consciousness of self is to accept it; to accept any thought that comes as part of ordinary thinking. This means that they should think about themselves and their illness *as much as the habit demands* and realize that *it is only a habit fostered by mental fatigue*. Once more I stress that the key to recovery is not in *forgetting* but in *no-longer-mattering*, and for this *time* must pass.

When the patient realizes that the intensity of his reaction is part of his sensitization and that if he accepts it and lets more time pass, those reactions will gradually become normal, then intense reaction can be borne more philosophically. This is sometimes called regaining one's balance and, as the Dutchman said to Vera Brittain, it takes time.

Recovery   43

❧

CHAPTER 3

Some Bewilderments Cleared Away

Over the last 20 years I have been treating nervously ill men and women in Australia, the United Kingdom, Canada and the United States by remote direction: recordings and regular journals in addition to my books. Some of the journals are included in Chapter Four.

Recently I asked some of these people if they had any further questions. I discuss these here and in Chapter Five.

FEELING LIKE PASSING OUT WHILE WASHING UP AT THE SINK

'When I get up in the morning I'm fine for a while and then, when I stand at the sink washing up, I get the feeling of going to pass out. My head gets tight and hot; my eyes won't focus properly and my neck tightens. Of course I take a tablet, although I always vow I won't.'

Sometimes a man or woman may feel comparatively well on rising and then the sight of some familiar thing (for the woman, quoted above, a sink full of dishes!) rings memory's bell and it tolls, 'Look out! You always feel faint here, remember? Watch out you don't fall! You could, you know!'

So stress comes and with it, tension: neck muscles contract; the head feels strange, light: eye muscles contract – the lens of the eye will not accommodate and sight is blurred. All because memory rang that wretched bell and tensed a body all too easily tensed.

Of course, with light-headedness comes fear of fainting, and although this woman says she's never actually fainted, she quickly presents herself with, 'What if?' So, more tension, more light-headedness, more defeat and probably poorly washed dishes. She wonders, 'Could there be something really wrong with my eyes? Am I going blind? and my neck ...?' When she begins to doubt, on comes more fear and the bind of extra tension. If only more doctors would explain symptoms more fully to patients whom they think neurotic, they would be surprised by the improvement in the patients.

If only this woman could understand how memory works and think 'What the heck! I can still manage to wash up even though I'm light-headed. I'm not going blind. My eye muscles will recover when I relax – anyhow, I can still wash up! So here goes!', how different she'd soon feel.

I'm not saying that the symptoms would all go quickly, they may not; but what a boost to her confidence to be able to work on, light-headed or not. And confidence brings relaxation and strength, so it wouldn't be long before she no longer noticed any light-headedness or blurred vision.

A good exercise for this woman would be to stand at the sink and see if she could make her symptoms more severe; even try to 'pass out' – this 'passing out' is not as easy as she thinks.

When she faces her symptoms this way, and is finally

prepared to accept and work with them there, there will be no need for a tablet and in time the sink would be once more only a sink.

JOINING THE WORLD AGAIN

'Your down-to-earth approach I find so helpful. You really do understand us. I have been receiving treatment from a young, well-meaning psychologist and although he was telling me to keep going out, he gave me no incentive to get going. He has been telling me that I have been hanging on to agoraphobia to keep me dependent on my daughter.

'I can't understand this as it's wonderful to be able to do things on my own and not have to ask my daughter to come with me.

'At last, with your help, after being shut in and depressed for weeks, I am walking into supermarkets, doing Christmas shopping. I'm part of life. After giving up a stressful job six months ago, I followed your advice and applied for a job as an assistant in a newspaper shop near home for a couple of hours a day. They took me on and, of course, I started worrying for fear I couldn't do it. My legs were like jelly, and my hands were shaking. I put on a bright smile and thought, "So what! They're not worried about me. I don't look any different." And I must say that, although feeling exhausted, by the end of the week I was so happy to collect that pay-packet.

'Another landmark was sitting through a church service. I hadn't been able to do this for a long time. I was up in the balcony, which made things worse, and I thought of all the people I'd have to pass if I wanted to go out. I felt uncomfortable after about an hour and took my coat off; but the panic didn't increase, although looking down made me feel quite dizzy. I just looked around and thought, "For all I know there could be some-one else here feeling like this!" I must say it was with some relief that I sang the last hymn. I feel as if I've joined the world again.'

RATHER WEEDY CREATURES?

'I resent the implication that I am a neurotic who can't cope in frightening, or tense situations. I cope, although frightened; which, of course, makes coping even more difficult. Am I not just a victim of particular circumstances, not a lesser human being? Or am I, as I so often feel, a rather weedy creature who should have learnt to be tougher?'

Most nervously ill people have been victims of particular circumstances. I quote a passage from Vicki Baume's autobiogra-phy: 'I know what I'm worth ... there are certain regions of fears in every one of us balanced by certain regions of courage. We are all constructed alike – 50 per cent hero, 50 per cent coward. As for myself, I am, and always was, a coward about noise and speed; I'm also frankly afraid of most mechanical contraptions including the telephone and the Mixmaster. They don't like me either and they could explode, couldn't they? Definitely I am a misfit for here and today.' (Vicki Baume was nearly 70 when she wrote this.) 'On the other hand, I bear up fairly well; I'm not afraid of the dark, of being left alone in the house, or of burglars, or of murderers and monsters – not a bit, if that doesn't sound too pompous.' She then goes on to say, 'My next great fear came in summer with the boom and hiss noise and flash of the fireworks and the hollering crowds on the Kaiser's birthday celebrations. I suppose this is where the fear of noise lodged in my bones and nerves.'

I liked her saying that we were 50 per cent coward and 50 per cent brave. I think we are. Maybe some of us are more afraid than others, some braver; but most of us belong to the 50/50 club.

We should not feel lesser human beings because we happen to be afraid in certain situations. Coping although frightened is true courage. As for being a weedy creature who should have learnt to be tougher, with a lot of practice in situations that frighten, we learn to be tougher, but this simply means learning how to cope with nervous reactions. It's as simple as that. When George Bernard Shaw was asked to take the chair at a British Association meeting, St John Irvine, who was present, said that Bernard Shaw's hand trembled so much with nervousness he could hardly sign the minutes.

Here again, acceptance and practice worked wonders. To quote St John again, nine years later Bernard Shaw was able to address the British Association with great aplomb.

Also, being at peace doesn't always mean having a peaceful body. We can be at peace while accepting an old rattling body. Indeed peace comes because we are *accepting while the body is rattling*. However, even with acceptance and practice, some of us may never know a completely calm body when under stress. The few who say they do are very lucky. Most of us have to work with the symptoms of stress present. I'd say we're all rather brave, not weedy, wouldn't you?

OBSESSION

A person tortured by an obsession is in my experience always capable of understanding – if only fleetingly – the truth about it. For example, a woman obsessed with the belief that her house was contaminated with germs could glimpse the truth while I explained to her that there were few dangerous germs present in any house. I had cultures made from smears taken from each of her rooms, from her refrigerator, tap water, around her drain pipes and so on and they were all negative.

When she saw these results she realized that her repeated cleaning (the refrigerator sometimes three times in one day!) was unnecessary.

Yet, as soon as she left me, her reaction to the thought of germs returned so strongly, she was once more caught up in the obsession.

That fleeting moment when she saw the truth behind her obsession, I call 'glimpsing'. I cure patients of obsession by teaching them to practise glimpsing regularly and often. To do this, they sit quietly (or stand, it doesn't really matter), think about their obsession and try to feel all the associated fear; then, while flooded in fear, *at that very moment*, to try to glimpse the truth behind the obsession, or simply to glimpse another point of view.

In the beginning, a mentally tired person (an obsession adds more fatigue to an already tired mind) may be able to glimpse only once or twice daily, but even one quick glimpse of the truth can expose the tricks that mental fatigue is playing and show that physical reaction to the obsession is severe because of sensitization (the constant tension from obsession can be very sensitizing) and not because of the importance, or truth, of the thought.

I have cured obsessions this way in people who have had years of unsuccessful orthodox treatment, including psychoanalysis, sedation, intravenous injection (e.g. Anafranil), narcoanalysis, electroconvulsive treatment (shock), hypnosis, group therapy and so on.

One woman, having had various treatments at a local psychiatric hospital over a period of nine years, was described to me in 1975 by her therapist as incurable. Later, at the same hospital, leucotomy was suggested. She refused.

I taught her to glimpse and she cured herself.

In November 1979, (after leucotomy had been refused and she had begun practising 'glimpsing') she wrote: 'The work you have done has been special. If it weren't for you a lot of us just wouldn't be here today, let alone happy to be here. You ask me if I have any questions left to ask you for your book. I have no more questions now, so I am going to repeat the question I asked you in 1975 while I was still ill. This is what I wrote then: "I have been a chronic severe obsessive for 17 years. As time has gone by I have got more and more obsessions and I have never got rid of any. Leucotomy has been discussed at the hospital but I would die first. Dr Weekes, can I ever get better?"'

She continued in her 1979 letter, 'Remember, that was the original question I asked you in 1975. It seems a long time ago now! As you know, with your help, I have been getting better ever since. I have found that with so many obsessions I have had to work on one at a time, using your method of glimpsing. I know that if one obsession is a strange silly thought, then they all are; but I find in practice I can't flay them all with one swoop. I work on one at a time; get it lukewarm, and then it goes. When they are white hot, if glimpsing is hard I just try to accept.

'I have now got to the stage where I can more or less count those I have left and they are only a few. They were innumerable. I shall get rid of these, I'm sure of it. But I know I can't do it any quicker than I am. I accept that too. Hasn't the outlook changed since Dr T. said I was incurable?'

One of her phobias was fear of falling pregnant. She became pregnant, resisted the suggestion of abortion on medical grounds, and is now the happy mother of a lovely young son.

In September-October 1983, I gave six talks on the BBC and this woman, Anne, was interviewed during these talks. During her last interview she was asked if she was happy. 'Oh, yes!' she said in her broad Yorkshire accent, 'You have to go through hell to know what heaven is! Oh, yes! I'm happy!'

Thank you, Anne, for coming on television and talking about yourself so openly for the sake of other suffering people. The letters that poured in during and after the talks (12,000 to the BBC apart from those that came to me) told how much people were helped.

SUPER-PANIC. HANGING ON TO A LAMPPOST FOR SUPPORT

'I have super-panics. I feel faint, dizzy, can't breathe properly and I'm sure I'm going to collapse. I've even hung on to lampposts for support. On top of this, I feel as though I'm "not there" and that I'm not going to come out of this terrible thing.

'How can I stop this sort of panic from coming on? I do *stay* on the bus, or walk down the street. I've tried to do what you've taught me, but when a panic is as bad as this, how can you expect people to let it come and carry on with what they're doing? Also, I'm drained when I've had an attack; I feel so weak and humiliated, how can I stay calm? I'm sure I'm about to die and I run for any escape I can see at the time.'

This is a striking example of what agoraphobia is all about. Every symptom this woman mentions comes from extreme fear, even terror, and she has put herself into this state because of her fear of the symptoms of fear. She is in a cycle of the symptoms of fear creating more fear.

Unfortunately a very brave woman has got herself into this impasse by thinking she was accepting when she was only putting up with. I appreciate fully how difficult becoming unafraid of panic is while its lash is so scorching. Small wonder so many despair. The lash can be so severe, the spirit seems to collapse beneath it.

While it is possible to take the severest flash without tranquillizers (and many do), I do not expect every sufferer to do so. A rest from practising with temporary tranqillization can give respite from suffering and help spirits rise until the sufferer is once more ready to face the tiger. After such respite he can let panic flash without crumpling so abjectly before it.

In my practice (I am now retired) I would ask such a person (usually on the telephone) to tell me what she believed I wanted her to do. I insisted that she put her idea of acceptance into her own words until I was sure she knew the difference between it and putting-up with.

I would ask her to try and *feel* acceptance right in her 'middle'. When she thought she did, I would say, 'Now walk down the street and hope you will panic so that you can practise accepting.'

So often a most relieved woman (or man) would return and say, 'I did it, doctor!' If she didn't 'make it' on that attempt, she usually did on the next. At least, we both persevered until she did.

I stress that there is great difference between temporarily taking tranquillizers for a short respite while in a state of supersensitization and depending on them as a permanent crutch.

Attacks of panic usually decrease in severity, and number, following a pattern. The person practising acceptance passes gradually from being terrified and dreading panic, to disliking it; then from disliking, to finding it no longer mattering. This does not mean that panic no longer comes. It takes time for no-longer-mattering to bring no panic. It is important to realize that panic can still flash and no longer matter. This is the beginning of recovery.

Please, please don't withdraw in terror from the symptoms of terror. There is no way out in withdrawal.

I know that some therapists either accompany, or provide people who will accompany, their agoraphobic patients until they can travel comfortably away from home. However, in my opinion, *these people are left vulnerable to returns of panic.*

I know mine is the hard way to be cured, but if we are to talk of permanent cure, then we talk of my way. *For permanent cure, a sufferer must learn to cope with his symptoms by learning to become unafraid of them.* He must not be led gently until he gets used to being away from the safety of home. *There is no permanent cure in getting used to being in a certain place so that panic does not come.*

If your heart fails when you read this, and you think that you could never practise what I teach, let it fail as much as it likes, but know that there is nobody who cannot practise this way if he makes up his mind to do it.

COPING WITH TREMBLING LEGS AND WEAKNESS, WHILE TALKING

A woman writing about this problem said, 'When there's nothing to sit on, and I must stand with jelly legs, how do I cope while I stand there shaking?'

The trembling legs and weakness are real. They are not imagined. After an asthmatic has had an injection of adrenalin, his legs tremble too, so that he has to sit, even lie down, for a few minutes. A nervously ill person's trembling and weakness have the same cause. Anxiety releases extra adrenalin. Once more, it's as simple as that.

However, although these trembling legs may seem as if they will give way, they don't. They could even climb steps. They will always support, so why add more anxiety – more adrenalin –

by anxiously wondering how much longer they will hold up, how much longer before the fainting comes!

Of course, even when recovered, during occasional stress, legs may seem to turn to jelly but, as I say in *Peace from Nervous Suffering*, jelly legs will always get you there if you let them.

CHANGE AND UNREALITY

'Why is it that if I visit someone and the decor is changed, or the building has been altered, even slightly (perhaps the inside of a bus has been painted a new colour), I immediately panic?'

Change, even slight, can act like a shock. It suddenly makes a nervously ill person aware of the outside world – as if it is demanding attention that he is reluctant to give. Also, if he has been using familiarity as a crutch, new decor could jolt sharply.

These are good experiences and should be welcomed until it no longer matters if the bus seems to be painted violet with yellow stripes!

THE MIND GOES BLANK, EVEN WHEN FEELING MUCH BETTER

Even when feeling better a mind can still suddenly seem to go blank. People like this complain that they can't remember the way they're supposed to be going, although they end by going the right way. They say that they feel as if they are in a dream, even when accompanied.

This is only the shadow of introspection – the result of living so much within themselves. It's not important; never be impressed by it. Wait and it will always pass. Of course, it passes more quickly if you don't add second-fear.

UNWANTED THOUGHTS

Never make the mistake of fighting to be rid of unwanted thoughts; relax towards them, let them come, take them with you – but WILLINGLY – and see even the most shocking for what they are: only thoughts.

If you fight to forget unwanted thoughts, or try to replace them with others, you make the unwanted thoughts too important so that forgetting becomes more and more difficult. It is always difficult to forget on command, especially if mentally tired.

A lot of practice at accepting and working while accompanied by upsetting thoughts may be needed to change them into 'just thoughts' with no upsetting reaction, holding no fear. Without fear, thoughts that once seemed to almost mesmerize can finally come to no longer matter. No-longer-mattering is the goal; *not* forgetting. One can never be sure of forgetting; memory is a great hoverer. However, if no-longer-mattering has been achieved through understanding and experience, one can depend on it with confidence.

Of course, from time to time, mattering will return. However, when not-mattering has been felt, if only for a moment, the mustard seed of confidence this brings will never actually disappear. As the sufferer pulls himself out of each setback by rediscovering not-mattering, it becomes in-built and comes quickly to his rescue whenever a setback threatens. The prize has been won.

I NO LONGER HAVE TO SIEVE THE JELLY

'It sounds ridiculous now, but obsessions are terrifying when you're having them. I can do anything today. I can even make jelly without putting it through a sieve for fear of it containing glass. One of the last things I lost was having to sieve the jelly. That's gone now; I get on with my baking. I've got about eight or nine tins of cakes in the pantry. I'm a good cook and now I can have my friends in and cook for them as they did for me. I want to be able to pay them back because of all the years of hospitality they gave me.

'They were wonderful. They did not understand obsessions but I said to them, "Just try and ignore them!" And they did. They didn't say a word. They were super friends.

'You know, I was ill for six years and I couldn't even go into the grocer's shop. I thought they'd have poisonous things on the shelves there – disinfectant and what not. I can go now and revel in it. I can walk out too, without checking everything. I can also go into the paper shop and the confectioner's. I haven't faced the chemist yet, but I know I'll be able to do that. I'm just wallowing in the relief at going into the other shops. I'll face the chemist soon. It's wonderful to be alive now. Thank you.'

PUNISHING THEMSELVES

Some nervously ill people complain that they 'seem to like punishing' themselves. One added, 'That is what nervous illness is all about, isn't it doctor?'

I have not yet met the nervously ill person who genuinely and deliberately adds to his illness simply to punish himself. His suffering may seem to be self-inflicted because, in his sensitized state, his thoughts, so often fearful, are followed so quickly by distressing symptoms that self-infliction seems the obvious interpretation. Indeed, some therapists believe this, even finding fantastic reasons for it, and they encourage their patients to do the same.

Self-punishment is only apparent; not real. When a nervously ill person says he seems to like punishing himself, he really means, 'Judging from my severe and swift reactions to my vaguest anxious thought, it seems as if I'm purposely punishing myself! I can think of no other explanation!' If such a person really liked punishing himself, he wouldn't be asking for help to stop it.

A TABLET BEFORE GOING OUT?

A woman wrote: 'Although I'm making great progress I still need to take a tablet most times before going out. Does it matter?'

There is a big difference between wanting and needing to take a tablet. I suspect that that woman wants to take a tablet because it gives her confidence. She thinks, 'I've had my pill so I'll be okay!' Many people, after swallowing a pill, are calm even before it hits their stomach.

That woman should have written, 'Although making great progress I still haven't enough courage to go out without taking a tranquillizer.' In fairness, I should add that I sometimes prescribe tablets for severely sensitized agoraphobic people to take occasionally before going out. So this woman should ask herself, 'Am I severely sensitized and genuinely in need of a tablet to calm me a little, or does taking a tablet simply give me confidence?' If she can answer honestly that the tablet only quietens the symptoms and does not altogether abolish them and that she must still practise accepting and seeing fear through, then she should take a tablet for the time being. If she has to ask herself, 'Should I, or shouldn't I, take a tablet?' the answer is, don't take it. Her need is psychological.

When I sometimes prescribe a tranquillizer for a severely sensitized person, I have first taught them how to go through panic *often enough* without tranquillization so that they know they can do it. With this experience, they understand that they are panic's master and can, while recovering, occasionally soften its blow with a mild tranquillizer – but never with heavy or constant tranquillization.

HOW MUCH SHOULD I DO?

'I'm confused about what I'm going through. I'm accustomed to going to Law School and working full-time at night. My health made me take a semester off. I'm wondering if, or when, I can get back into the swing of things?'

One of the hurdles obstructing some people recovering from nervous illness is to decide how much of their fatigue is normal everyday fatigue – the sort they felt before they were ill – and how much is due to lingering illness. In other words, they wonder if they should treat their fatigue with respect 'for fear of making it worse', or if they should work on despite it? They are confused.

They need not fear physically overtiring themselves providing they are prepared to accept its effects optimistically. If they work hard one day, they may feel some nervous symptoms more acutely the next, but if they accept this willingly, the symptoms will soon calm. Action and achievement are more important than inaction, 'for fear of overdoing it'. With action accompanied by willing acceptance of any fatigue that may follow, one gradually becomes confident. Working physically, even 'overdoing it', will not damage nerves; it's the tension from anxiety that sensitizes and brings fatigue.

This advice also applies to working hard mentally. It's the anxiety accompanying the working that tires, rarely the actual work. The person who has to take a semester off because of the effects of work, will be apprehensive at the thought of beginning work again. He should understand and expect this and not try to be too stoic. He should let himself be apprehensive and understand that in the circumstances this is to be expected. Fear and lack of confidence will certainly make concentrating and remembering difficult in the beginning; he should expect and understand this. And if he must re-read (perhaps many times) a sentence, or a paragraph, before fully understanding it, then he must re-read: but *willingly*.

Gradually he will find that studying and remembering will become easier; confidence will return. He will achieve all this by first accepting apprehension, loss of confidence, even muzzy head, and working willingly and quietly determinedly *with them all present*.

ENJOYING LIFE TO THE FULL

'After watching you for several weeks on BBC Television I am writing a long overdue letter of gratitude to you. I bought both your books five years ago after hearing about you on the radio. I discovered that I was one of the people who was going to find it extremely difficult to put your teaching into practice, but I persevered and now from being extremely ill (worse after spending a short time in hospital) and suffering from agoraphobia and all the accompanying symptoms, I can today enjoy life to

the full and live with, and for, my family who were very support-
ive through a very trying time. I'm now holding down a job
which seemed an impossibility five years ago. I still have the
habit of memory and flashbacks to the old ways but I practise
your method and I always come through. I sometimes think that
even today somebody, somewhere, is going to wake up sensitized and be bewildered and not know what to do about it. Your
work must never be forgotten and it must go on.'

WAKING EARLY: THE MORNING'S
KNIFE EDGE

The upsetting symptoms that can come to a nervous person
on waking have been called the startle syndrome. Sensitized
nerves can be startled by the slight shock of waking even though
the waker may not recognize any shock. Also the sufferer may go
to bed at night feeling relieved and peaceful, only to wake the
next morning and feel the same old thumping heart, tingling
body and that old familiar feeling of foreboding. The optimistic
feelings of the night before seem to have little influence on the
mood of the next morning. The feeling of foreboding may seem
so real that the sufferer may search for some impending trouble
to explain it. Also, when he first wakes, his nerves may be so
'raw' he feels as if he is balanced on a knife's edge. This is a legacy from the tension of the previous days. Even when the sufferer
is almost recovered, some slight renewed stress may bring on
again a few mornings of startle and foreboding. Why worry!

Getting up, going to the bathroom, making a hot drink may
be enough to break the spell. At least the sufferer should let
the feelings come; not try to push them away. He should relax
toward them.

Sometimes, if he continues to lie in a troubled half-sleep, the feeling of being on the knife's edge is accentuated. That half-sleep leaves him vulnerable to little shocks from outside noises and each shock can 'twang' his nerves – hence the knife's edge! It is better to wake right up, move about, perhaps read, than lie in that perplexed, troubled 'raw' state.

ALL SO QUIET IN THOSE EARLY HOURS – SO STILL

To a nervously ill person who wakes in the very early hours, the quietness can seem threatening; even the sound of the early morning garbage van is welcome. At least someone is alive! And, oh!, the relief of hearing movement in the house, especially the rattling of cups and saucers!

I once mentioned early morning quietness to a patient from the country. She laughed and said, 'Oh, doctor, you've obviously never lived in the country! You should just hear the animals at our place and the sound of heavy boots stomping around the kitchen at the crack of dawn!' Perhaps the sound of heavy boots is comforting someone at this moment.

Noises that come regularly at a set time – for example once or twice a week – can be a yardstick to gauge progress or lack of it. Every Tuesday when the garbage van calls, the rattling cans can bring hope, or the despair of 'another bloody Tuesday!'

Sometimes the early morning waker can be so anxious to return to sleep and blot out those hours of waiting, she becomes wider and wider awake.

In my opinion there is a stage in nervous illness when an early morning sedative may be necessary. It may be better, if the sufferer is agitated, to shut out those early hours of lonely suffering, than to have him exhaust himself trying to live through them – accepting one minute, being overwhelmed the next.

However, waking later – at about 5 o'clock or after – is no time for a pill. At this time it's better to wake right up, listen to the radio, read, get a hot drink. Taking a sleeping pill at 5 or after can make the body feel even heavier when trying later to heave it off the bed to face another day.

Some nervously ill people expect to sleep the night through, irrespective of the time they retire. One woman said, 'I had a bad night last night, doctor!' She'd gone to bed at 7 the previous night, so by 3 o'clock she'd already had eight hours of sleep – everybody's quota. Her problem was that by 7 she had to fight to keep awake. It's so easy for friends to say, 'Stay up until late; then you won't wake so early!' This isn't always true. Eyes that are sleepy early in the evening can pop open widely as soon as they later hit the pillow; their owner may then lie agitatedly for hours and end by taking a sleeping pill after all.

If a severely fatigued person comes to me with a problem of early waking because of retiring too early, or because of sleeping during the day, I advise him to sleep when he feels like it, whatever the hour. As little as one hour's sleep in the afternoon can freshen enough to help get through the rest of the day and does not always interfere with sleeping at night.

It is essential at the stage of severe sensitization to get as much sleep as possible. When a sensitized person is severely fatigued, he needs sleep, not further agitation.

DRIVING A CAR AND AGORAPHOBIA

One woman said that in a car she could talk her way through a crisis without anyone seeing her – she could say my words out aloud to herself. She admitted that in some ways travelling in a car and perhaps taking a friend was a disadvantage because she came to rely on them both too much. She said, 'Should I start again, the right way, alone without the car? I need you personally to tell me, so that I can drum what you say into myself over and over again. Is my car an advantage or is it a disadvantage?'

Driving a car while recovering from agoraphobia is neither an advantage nor a disadvantage; everything depends on attitude not on the car. Everything depends on whether the agoraphobic uses the car as a prop or not. This woman is using it as a prop. In her heart she knows she must do without props. In her favour, at least she recognizes this. But now she wants to use my words as ejector and prop. I want her to prop *herself* up, doing the things she fears the way I have taught her. She must look for the strength *within herself* to do just that. Strength is always there if we truly want it.

At this stage, she must *not* try to find courage in a command from me! At this stage, after relying so much on car and friend, she must search for her own precious (there is no other word for it) mustard seed of courage and then: Onward! Through!

TRAVELLING FAST IN A BUS OR TRAIN

Allow your body to travel with the moving vehicle, go with the movement, don't tense against it.

If you stand at a busy street and watch and listen to the heavy traffic go by, it usually seems excessively fast and noisy. However if you are actually driving a car in that traffic, you are much less aware of speed or noise, because you are going forward with the movement of the car; you are part of the traffic. So, if travelling in a fast bus or train, or any other fast vehicle, take a deep breath, let it out slowly and let yourself move forward, with the vehicle, don't tense yourself against the movement. Loosen, let go. If you do this, the movement will not seem so fast.

JUST 'A TOUCH' OF AGORAPHOBIA

In practice I never use the word agoraphobia, so my patients have never felt labelled. In my opinion, labelling phases of nervous illness can be dangerous. For example, a woman telephoned today saying she'd had a nervous breakdown for three years and that while that had been difficult enough, one of the doctors at the hospital had labelled her 'possibly schizophrenic'. She now felt such intense anxiety she didn't know how she could live with it. That careless labelling had presented her with a burden, almost too heavy to bear.

Agoraphobia is no more than one aspect of an ordinary anxiety state. A person in an anxiety state may have rapidly beating heart, sweating hands, may feel weak, giddy and have flashes of panic which grow worse if he is out where he thinks he may be trapped, cannot escape and so may end by making a fool of himself before other people. Hence, he may avoid going out and mixing with people, especially in a confined situation (public hall, church and so on).

In my opinion this is the basis of most agoraphobia and is a natural sequence to an anxiety state. And since it is possible to be in a mild or severe anxiety state, it's also possible to have mild or severe agoraphobia. For example, some days a person may feel well enough to go out alone, even to the supermarket, and yet on another day feel unable to face the front door. That is mild agoraphobia. A severe agoraphobic never goes out alone and may even refuse to go if accompanied.

There are certainly grades of the agoraphobic phase of an anxiety state.

OUT OF THE BOG

Many people trying to recover from nervous illness have the feeling that they must struggle up, up, out of some depth, almost as if they have to drag themselves out of some kind of bog to finally feel *on top* of things; on the same level as life around them. For example, when they hear of a friend going on holiday they think of him as being 'on the same level!' as the place he is going to – he has only to pack a case and be off! Whereas, for the sufferer, going for a holiday would seem like going to somewhere in the sky above: far, far out of reach.

He does not understand that he feels like this because, to face travelling, he would have to come 'out of himself', 'up from the depths'; up, out of his grey world of introspection. And it *is* a grey world. The sun may shine, but his mind is so dulled by tiring, endless, anxious introspection, his eye muscles so tensed by anxiety, that the world may actually look grey.

Also, to simply be on the same daily level as other people (with no thought of a holiday) seems to require energy he thinks he will never have. The bog is so deep and clinging!

Time, more time and acceptance make the impossible gradually possible. The bog becomes dry land.

CAN NERVOUS ILLNESS CAUSE FITS?

'Can a nervously ill person, when in a panic, have a fit? When I was rushed to hospital with thrombosis in 1950, they said I had

had a fit. Actually I had been on barbiturates for many years, five or six a day, and my GP said that my fit was due to the sudden withdrawal of these tablets. You see, I didn't tell the nursing staff that I was taking them. I hope my doctor was right. Even today, I am petrified of the word 'fit' and wish people wouldn't use it lightly. Even to write it is making my stomach churn now.'

Withdrawal from heavy doses of some tranquillizers, especially barbiturates and benzodiazapines (valium and its relatives), can cause fits. Nervous illness itself does *not* cause fits. The word 'fit' upsets many people, not only the writer of that letter. Understanding clearly what a fit is could help to lose fear of it. When we look at fear squarely it usually becomes less fearful. Fear doesn't like being looked at! Although this woman now shrinks from the thought of it, I doubt if she has seen a fit. The sooner she learns to face the thought of it without fear, the sooner she will be free to move without fear.

When we want to move our body, our brain sends messages to the muscles concerned. In epilepsy this part of the brain sometimes triggers messages without conscious direction and the muscles dutifully respond. An epileptic woman is most vulnerable pre-menstrually, when her brain is irritated by the retention of fluid due to hormonal imbalance. Regulating fluid and salt intake at that time may be enough to stop the fits.

It's not pleasant to watch someone having a fit but as usual familiarity brings tolerance. During one of these spontaneous bursts of muscle movement (that's all a fit is), arms and legs flay about. At the same time, the victim loses consciousness, may wet his pants and perhaps bite his tongue. Is that so terrible? Many of us do some of these gymnastic feats at some time. The big difference is that the person fitting does them all at the same time. Look at it that way.

If you should ever see someone taking a fit (after all Caesar, St Paul, Alexander the Great, even Mohammed took them, so why not someone you know?), instead of running away, stay and help. Remove any obstacle which he may hit and so hurt himself.

As mentioned earlier, nervous illness does not cause fits.

FEAR-FLASHES

'I'm not quite sure what is making me afraid, but I have fear-flashes when I look at, or think, certain things; for example, I am afraid I may harm someone. Some days I may just have to look at someone, or touch something, to have that reaction. The picture may seem so clear, it blocks out everything else. This really frightens me.'

So many lives have been spoiled by a sensitized body's too acute reaction to some fearful thought. Without such exaggerated reaction, this woman could have reasoned with herself and been able to think, 'Of course I wouldn't harm anyone! How silly!' And that would be that. But when thoughts are accompanied by a strong stab of physical fear, the victim may be shocked and bewildered. At such a moment, it is natural to take the thoughts seriously and believe that perhaps he, or she, really could harm someone and so perhaps, develop an obsession about it, as this woman has.

If only such people could understand that the thought frightens them only because of their body's sensitized reaction to it and not because it is a real threat. If only they could see the strength of their reaction as part of a physical (sensitized) state, unrelated to truth, and pass through the flash and continue on with the job on hand, how many lives could be saved from exhausting misery! I recently spoke on BBC television about some nervously ill people fearing that they would harm others and received a letter from a woman who, for 30 years, has had this fear. Simply hearing me explain it had freed her. So many years wasted for lack of simple explanation.

FRIGHTENED OF BEING ALONE

An American woman wrote, 'In the summer I am pretty much okay. I can put the kids on the bike or play with them outside. I can talk with my neighbours, but something awful happens to me come November when I know I will be stuck inside the house for most of the winter.

'My husband takes our only car for the day and I haven't driven out of our small town alone since I got sick. I had so many bad attacks in the car, memory of them is holding me back. In your book, you say pull the car over and wait. I've never been able to do that. The longer I sit the worse I get, so I drive quickly in a terrible state – anything to get home.

'When I am in the house this time of year, I feel my illness hovering over my shoulder and I panic at the thought of it. My children need me; there will be no-one to care for them if I weren't here – I need to be well. I don't know what to do or why I feel like this. My days are lonely and boring. Why am I so dependent on other people? I can do just anything if someone is with me, even drive the car. To sit here a week alone seems impossible.

'Sometimes I feel I am losing my mind because I can't stand my feelings or see a solution. I just know I don't want to be alone.'

To bear aloneness contentedly – especially during long, dark, winter days – one has to be very much at peace within oneself. Even those at peace depend on being occupied during the winter. But they have the advantage of being calm enough to sit down and plan for winter days; when the woman who wrote that letter sits and thinks of the long, dark days ahead, she becomes confused by fear and dread. Housework certainly may not hold enough interest, and small children can be demanding and frustrating.

It's important to be able to tolerate being alone, otherwise one can spend a lifetime running away from oneself. Here is an exercise for this woman: when the children are bedded down for their morning sleep, she should sit and face the silence, not shrink away from it; she should drench herself in self-awareness. She will find that after a while, her mind will begin to wander. She will think of some job that needs doing; her thoughts will flicker out to the laundry, into the bedroom or perhaps she will just watch the trees in the garden. She should repeat this exercise whenever she feels overpowered by that moment of aloneness that is so difficult to live through.

When she is prepared to face the quietness in this way, she will find that the hovering monster will gradually stop hovering. She will lose her fear of being alone and it is this, her fear, that brings the under-current of tension she dreads.

When she can pass through that moment by facing it and being ready to be swamped by it – not withdrawing from it – she will find she will be able to sit and read a book contentedly, pick up a piece of sewing and, more important still, will be able to plan for the winter days ahead. She will be able to live in the moment, not in fear of it.

OLD AGE OR NERVOUS ILLNESS?

'How does one cope with getting old and at the same time, with the remnants of nervous illness? My illness seems to be taken over by the feelings of advancing age. I'm making no real progress that I can see because of not being able to cope with work or pleasure, or even with a journey by car to go on holiday. And yet I've lived through 15 years of nervous illness! This feeling of great effort takes me back years to the days when I was first going downhill. Perhaps this is why I feel that the cause is now not so much illness as old age?

'With the book (*Self Help for Your Nerves*) you have given me, I was able to cope with my illness and I do lead a reasonable life, but I want to enjoy life to make up for the years wasted. Others live and grow old, but I feel that we phobics gave up living when we became ill and yet, when we recover, we expect to carry on just where we left off, perhaps years ago. How can I come to terms with all this?

'The things about the house and garden that I used to do, even when I felt bad, I can't get the strength to do now. If I make myself do them I get tired with aches and pains and it doesn't seem worthwhile. I'm sure there's a link between feeling this way now and the years spent in nervous illness while life was hell. I'm sure I'm feeling the result of this more now because I'm older.

'I'm rambling on about the same thing, but I'm not alone in this experience; many of my contacts have the same problem. I've been asked, "Has the fight been worth it?" If I go down again now, I feel I'll never be able to fight back. It has all taken too long. Is it my age that makes me feel unable to cope now, or the memory of my past illness?'

Your tiredness is probably more a legacy of illness than of age, although you don't say how old you are – you talk only of 'advancing' years. Naturally resilience and energy decrease with age and with them go motivation and, so often, interest. Usually the change is gradual, whereas I suspect that you feel old suddenly.

Prolonged nervous illness brings fatigue of the spirit and, in my opinion, this is probably your main trouble. While you were struggling to recover earlier, it was not so much that you were younger as that you had a goal and hope – two prime motivators. Now you are not only tired by the struggle, you have also lost confidence *because you know you are growing old* and therefore think that feeling tired is irrevocable.

If you have the courage to replace despair with fresh hope and willingness to accept once more, you will gradually feel strength return. Peace of mind is a wonderful healer and you apparently have little of that now.

Your question has been asked of me many times. I have found that if the questioner stops trying to fathom how much fatigue is the result of nervous illness and how much of old age, and instead does what he can within the limits of his present strength without thrashing himself too severely with doubt and bewilderment, he is surprised how much he can gradually do. Our bodies have great recuperative powers if we remove tension – even in our eighties. I have proved this on myself.

Also, many nervously ill people do not lead active lives during their illness and suffer from lack of exercise – muscles become flabby and legs tire so easily that sitting or lying, instead of walking, is a constant temptation.

Even the memory of tiredness can bring a feeling of fatigue, and as for the thought of facing 'it all' again ...! Small wonder you baulk at it.

My advice is: don't look for progress; take each day as it comes, doing what must be done without asking too many questions. Don't protest too vehemently; that wastes strength.

Be sure you eat enough nourishing food and are not taking tranquillizers habitually or a too heavy dose of sleeping pills at night. As we grow older we tolerate drugs poorly; small doses can have big effects. Also, if you are only picking at food, I suggest a moderate dose of vitamins.

Once more, acceptance; but with a fresh heart.

AN ON-AND-OFF AFFAIR

'After I first saw you, the level of my recovery became good enough for me to carry on in an important job in the Public Service for 10 more years. Then I thought: I've handled this well so far, so I can retire!

'The reason I could manage so well was that although I sometimes still felt lousy in the mornings and struggled to work, the moment I became engrossed in work – especially if it was a research project – I found myself feeling normal. And then sometimes, I had only to become aware of feeling good when I immediately felt awful again! That's the way it goes! It's an on-and-off affair, isn't it? Why?'

Finding oneself suddenly well like this can be a shock: a shock that brings apprehension and, apprehension soon brings a return of nervous symptoms. The switch from feeling well to suddenly feeling symptoms again can be so upsetting, bewildering, that the nervously ill person can become almost afraid to feel well. One man said, 'I'd rather stay down all the time, than go through this yo-yo business!'

The sufferer must learn to pass through those moments of flash-fear and not let them throw him off balance. On, on, on! Through the flash, through any return of symptoms; through that pain of contracting heart; through and on! Recovery always lies AHEAD, however painful the moment.

AFRAID TO FEEL ORDINARY FEELINGS

During recovery, a nervous person may be afraid to feel ordinary feelings. His emotions have been exaggerated for so long he feels lost, not knowing what to feel. He may think, 'Is what I feel now normal? What *is* normal?'

There are so many hazards on the way to recovery. Small wonder acceptance of all strange feelings is the answer. What else could it be?

HYPOCHONDRIA

A nervously fatigued, or nervously ill person, is suggestible: a pain here, a weakness there, is enough to convince him that he has some strange disease – so often, multiple sclerosis. Formerly he would have worried little about these symptoms, or would have seen his doctor without too much concern.

In my opinion, few nervously ill people are true hypochondriacs. They are simply people who are tired of being ill and are so sensitized, they feel they can't bear the extra strain of worrying about new physical symptoms. They should not be ashamed if they feel they need to visit their doctor frequently, to get relief from worry. They should explain to their doctor that in their present state they cannot avoid noticing every new symptom that appears; that their nerves are reacting in an exaggerated way and they need the peace they hope his explanation will bring. They are not true hypochondriacs.

WHEN THE AEROPLANE DOORS CLOSE

'What should I do, or not do, when the aeroplane doors close? I would like to be able to accept an invitation to visit friends in the United States; that is an eight-hour flight. So please could you help me?'

To sit in tension trying not to panic while the aeroplane doors close could mean trying to sit on panic for the rest of the journey. The anxious traveller should be prepared to panic and think, 'Okay, I'm going to panic, so here goes! Let it come!' His very acceptance (real acceptance, not just lip service!) will take the edge off panic. But while he panics he mustn't watch to see if the edge has gone! That's not accepting.

If he does find the courage to take that journey and is willing to panic – the way I teach: loosening the body, letting it slump in the seat, breathing in deeply and out slowly, without withdrawing in panic from panic – he will find that he will gradually become interested in what goes on around him more than in remembering to panic. Actually, the inside of a jet is rather like a busy hotel dining room – so much going on down those aisles.

As I say so often, it's contemplation that is the killer! Anticipating the journey can be worse than making it, but how many have the courage to prove that?

When the frightened person thinks of travelling, he imagines the entire journey being spent in continuous panic. It isn't like that. Once he accepts the closed doors, he may find a certain elation – he has 'made it', is actually there, in the seat! He may even talk to his neighbour, watch a movie. Time does pass.

Instead of thinking of seven hours (the journey from London to New York) at a stretch, he should divide the hours into halves and see each half hour through. Also, on a long journey he may feel drowsy and sleep through some of the time.

Readers may think, 'Not me! I'd never sleep inside an aeroplane!' They could be surprised.

Some aeroplane companies have special courses for people afraid of plane travel. They claim to have good results. However, an agoraphobic's fear differs from the usual fear of plane travel; he is not afraid so much of having an accident or the feeling of flying. He is afraid of being hemmed in, unable to escape from his own reactions; afraid of the hell he imagines he could create for himself.

One woman, afraid of panicking in a plane, always carried valium tablets (just in case). On a particular journey, she managed to see the doors close without having to take a tablet, but when the person beside her started to get worked-up, she felt her own panic rising and succumbed to a valium. Within a few minutes she was calm. It wasn't until that night that she discovered she'd taken a Vitamin B tablet, not a valium. From then on she travelled pill-less.

If you want to travel without the crutch of a tablet, you can. However severe your panic, simply sit back and roll with the punches. Let come what will. Whatever comes won't kill you, and you certainly *won't* have hysterics and go rushing down the aisle as you've been imagining all these weeks. Watch the doors close and let the panic rip; but see it through the right way! That means not withdrawing from it in panic. It means understanding that it is no more than an electrical flash; so see it to the end and don't let an electrical flash stop you seeing your friends in Arkansas! The person who sees panic through is so much more confident, so much more recovered, than the one who sits on panic trying to think of other things 'to stop panic coming'. Bon voyage!

THE FED-UP FAMILY

'I hide your books under the bed now. My family has become allergic to my complaints. They're so fed up with hearing, "As Dr Weekes says ...!" I hope you won't be upset by this, doctor. Your books are a great help to me.'

Few people want to hear about another's suffering – especially nervous suffering – and families in particular become gradually browned off. This does not mean that they are necessarily unsympathetic; their own nerves begin to suffer from tension – and living with a nervously ill person means living under tension, especially when spirits rise with the sufferer's improvement and sink with the disappointment of a setback. Few families can survive cheerfully for long, so don't blame your family too much. And yet, to have someone to go to for a little understanding is one of the nervously ill person's dearest wishes. However, as I have said so often, nervous illness can be a lonely business.

GRATITUDE

'To show you how much I have recovered: I went to the hospital this week to a conference on psychiatry and I sat in front of about 50 doctors and answered their questions about my illness. My mouth felt dry and my arms tingled, but I managed to survive this nerve-racking ordeal. In fact, I rather enjoyed educating the audience. Again I say: thank you for making this all possible, doctor.'

RESTING ON THE BED IN THE DAYTIME

'I get a lot of help from your books, but I can hardly agree when you say, "Keep off that bed in the daytime!". I get so very tired doing my level best to carry on with every nerve crying out loudly to rest. Someone rang me just now and the shock of the telephone nearly killed me. I have suffered all my life with nerves and some of your advice has helped a lot, except that bit about keeping off the bed in the daytime. Oh dear, I thought I could cope with it better. I was going to tell my doctor how much you'd helped me until now! If you could possibly write and explain what you mean by keeping off that bed in the daytime, it would certainly be a help.'

This woman is 70 and recently had an accident. Her wounds became infected and she was in hospital for weeks and had to return there for further treatment. Of course, she should have rested on the bed or couch in the daytime. This is an example of how careful and explicit a doctor should be when speaking or writing. I thought I was careful but I wasn't thinking of victims of accidents.

Others have been puzzled by my statement about keeping off the bed in the daytime. When I made that statement I was thinking of nervously depressed people who would take to bed as a refuge and lie and brood on their illness, convinced that they hadn't the strength to get up and do anything about it. Also, I thought of the nervously ill person who would lie and worry about his problems and rise later feeling worse than when he lay down. A pillow makes a too encouraging nest for a head full of worry.

Of course, people who know they will benefit from daytime rest (as this woman obviously did) should take it. No question.

Why be alarmed by any strange feeling during nervous illness? Some are bound to come. A baby learning to walk must surely feel strange as he notices how tall the chairs, and especially father, seem. However, he goes on and eventually walks, accepting their towering height. That's how we grow up.

A sensitized, nervous person should learn the lesson of accepting strangeness, any strangeness that is nervous, *until it no longer matters*. There will always be tall buildings, they'll never shorten to oblige us; so practise looking at them with acceptance as you breath in and out deeply and slowly.

Take a brave, especially relaxed look at them as you breath out. What the heck!

WHAT CAUSES SETBACKS?

A setback usually comes in two stages: first, a sufferer's sensitized reaction to some disturbing circumstance or memory, and then his alarm at the return of the old familiar nervous symptoms.

While some sensitization lingers, stress can trigger the return of many, if not all, of the old symptoms. If the sufferer understands and accepts this, they gradually subside. However, if he becomes afraid and tense and thinks, 'Here I go again! I'm going to slip right back!' and stays afraid, he opens the door to setback. It's the second fear – the fear of setback itself that he adds – that can entrench him in setback.

A sensitized body can continue to react intensely and swiftly to stress even when the sufferer understands and has reached a stage where the symptoms no longer upset him. Physical recovery so often lags behind understanding and acceptance, that it's good to be prepared for an occasional flash of sensitivity; being prepared is the best defence. More time must pass; the way is always on and through, always onward.

With enough practice going into, and out of, setback, setbacks may threaten, even come, but they no longer frighten, and when a setback no longer frightens, it passes very quickly. Indeed it is no longer a setback – it is not even a halt – it's simply an accepted, even expected, experience on the way to recovery.

HOW SHORT IS A SHORT ILLNESS?

If a sufferer has had no satisfactory treatment for nervous illness, I would call one year of illness short. Illness for a few months would be very short. If a sufferer is having adequate treatment then, in my opinion, three months would be the average time for recovery. I have had patients recover after one interview. Although rare, this has happened.

HOW MUCH SHOULD I DO?

So much depends on the depth of fatigue. A nervously ill person may feel so exhausted when he finally decides to get off the bed and face recovery that he may need physical support – an arm to lean on. However, with determination and the right kind of effort, nervous fatigue can pass surprisingly quickly – within three or four weeks. Having some kind of occupation, fortified by acceptance, restores strength faster than 'resting on the couch'.

Also, a nervously ill person who, on rising, feels that he has not the strength even to make the bed, will often find that by the end of the day's work he has more energy than when he first got up. Physical work exhausts less than does anxious introspection.

Don't worry about how much you should do, simply go and do what has to be done, willingly; rest at intervals, again willingly, and do not feel anxiously guilty about 'all that work piling up'.

Never push yourself to prove how much you can do; pushing means tension. On the other hand, don't go round the house working at a snail's pace for fear of 'pushing'. It really doesn't matter whether you work quickly, or slowly, as long as you work with willing acceptance of how you feel and of how much you have left undone.

STRENUOUS SPORT WHILE DEPLETED?

A man asked this question.

I have yet to meet the depleted person who wants to play strenuous sport. However, I have seen some young people who thought they were too weak to leave the beds on which they had been lying for years, play tennis after only a few weeks of the right treatment.

One man, more or less confined to bed for nine years, said he felt so ill he hadn't the strength to read my book, *Self Help for Your Nerves* (called *Hope and Help for Your Nerves* in America); a friend read it to him. And yet, after listening to these readings and then practising walking with golfsticks as crutches, he was playing tennis within six weeks. His story was published in the *New York Times Magazine* around Christmas 1977. One finds strength quicker when active than when lying on the couch waiting for it to come.

I encourage patients to be active, but before I would advise strenuous sport I would need to examine the adventurer. Swimming I advise because it need not be strenuous and if in salt water is especially soothing to those trying to come off tranquillizers. It brings its own sedation.

Also, during the agitation that can accompany drug withdrawal, exercises help 'let off steam', and I recommend them.

OUR POWER TO ADAPT

A woman recovering from nervous illness went to stay with some friends at the seaside. When she first saw the cottage her heart sank. It was weatherboard and old and reminded her of similar cottages in which she had lived years ago when young and poor. The memory was depressing and she was further depressed when she remembered she was committed to stay for a month!

However, she let the first shock pass and found, after a few days, that she quite enjoyed resting on the sunny veranda and that the store on the corner was handy; the woman next-door, kind; and that the linoleum on the floor and the ugly old-fashioned dresser in the kitchen no longer bothered her. The disliked kitchen became a warm, welcoming place.

We should always remember to let the first shock pass and never run away too soon. Our power to adapt is irrepressible if we give it a chance.

WHEN IS A PERSON 'TOO OLD' FOR RECOVERY?

Much depends on circumstances and unfortunately, when a person is old, these may not be very encouraging. An old person may feel himself a burden to family and friends – to those friends left! Having to put on an act before the family accentuates loneliness, weariness, even apathy. It's sometimes difficult to decide how much weariness and depression are due to circumstances and how much to old age. One man, always tired, always lying down, was found to be diabetic; with treatment he now spends hours in the garden. He said, 'I could never work out what was natural tiredness for my age and what was an underlying illness!'

Many people in their seventies have this same puzzle. I am so often asked, 'Is it my nerves or just my age, doctor?' An old person should be examined regularly by a caring doctor. Age itself is no bar to recovery from 'nerves'. So much of the trauma in growing old is psychological. One has but to see the effect of turning 70 on some people to understand the power of suggestion. A friend said to me, 'I was all right when I was 69. The minute I turned 70 I felt old!' If we could grow old like other animals without knowing our age, there would be many more healthier, fewer depressed, old people.

Of course recovery is helped by finding an interesting occupation, particularly in the company of other people. Finding an interesting occupation is the biggest stumbling block to recovery for young people; for old people it's like searching for the crock of gold at the end of the rainbow. So easy to prescribe; so hard to find.

A friend told me about her father, aged 92, for whom they were trying to find some new occupation. They made one offer and he said 'I don't want to do that! I want something with some future to it!'

And how's this for spirit? A woman wrote, 'I'm extraordinarily better and count myself cured. I'm 89 and have to wear a hearing aid. Most people have to wear theirs during the day, but I have to wear mine at night as well. I feel I must hear the clock ticking. I panic if I can't, so I have two clocks to be on the safe side. Also I can't sleep in the dark without a night-light.

'When I think of the hours and days I walked about the

streets because I couldn't stay in the house, it seems a small thing to ask. I owe everything to your kind help. My lip-reading teacher had a sudden attack from working too hard. She is having a year off. I lent her your book and she has found it a great help and is much better.'

So here's a woman of nearly 90 asking about complete cure. That should cheer on the babes of 70. But what is there for her to be 'really cured of'? – a ticking clock and a little night-light. Surely she is entitled to both.

When old, it's so easy to be apprehensive at night. During the day, with familiar homely things around, apprehension dims but in the dark aloneness at night, the ticking clock and the little light mean that home is still there even in the dark.

AGORAPHOBIA AND LIVING IN A CITY LIKE NEW YORK

'I developed agoraphobia about 10 years ago when New York started to deteriorate so badly. I don't travel in the subway or walk around at night for fear of being mugged. I really feel this should be included in any talk about agoraphobia.

'Of course books and articles are now being written about agoraphobia; in fact it is the "in" thing. I don't find that very funny. To me the reality is too painful. Agoraphobia should not be a cocktail or TV session curiosity, should it?'

To be afraid of moving around in a big city after dark, or travelling in the subway, because of legitimate fears of being mugged, is not agoraphobia. While a person can circulate freely when in an area safe from mugging, can go on holiday, attend meetings and so on, he is not agoraphobic. In a smaller, safer town he would probably travel everywhere without fear.

It is true that there is much talk about agoraphobia today. Before the early sixties few had heard of it and later, when they did, the idea of a man or woman (usually woman) staying at home for years for fear of travelling away from home – even being afraid to go to the postbox to post a letter – intrigued so many people, it soon became a conversation piece and a media pet. Better to have people interested and even gossiping about agoraphobia than being ignorant of its existence.

Some of the amused people were not so flippant when they suddenly discovered the cause of Aunt Ethel's persistent refusal to go on a holiday with them, or a friend's persistent refusal to dine at a certain restaurant. These are real examples. After being on television or radio, I sometimes found a member of the staff waiting for me at the studio exit. They would confide secretly about some member of their family or friend who, they now discovered, was agoraphobic.

In one city, the driver of my car invariably came with me while I broadcast and stood in the shadows in the studio. I said, 'Bill, you don't have to accompany me while I talk!' He answered, 'Oh, yes I do, doctor! I understand now what's been wrong with my wife these last three years and I'm learning how to help her. She's listening in too!'

Better small-talk than no talk.

AN ORIGINAL CAUSE

If, by finding an original cause, a nervously ill person loses his fear, then he can be cured because losing fear is simply another way of describing recovery. However, cure only occasionally lies in finding an original cause, because, even with cause found, nervous symptoms so often remain. Sensitization has the last word, and finding an original cause does not necessarily desensitize. The sufferer may have become afraid of physical nervous symptoms.

In my opinion, in the past there has been too much emphasis on curing by finding possible subconscious causes; thankfully, today therapists are more willing to admit that an original cause may no longer be working, may even be unimportant, at the time when the patient comes for help. Great relief to us all!

THAT NIGGLY FEELING: COULD THE SYMPTOMS RETURN?

A man wrote, 'Although I feel I'm almost cured, will I always have that niggly fear that all the symptoms could come back?'

The niggly fear will linger so long as the thought of a return of symptoms brings apprehension. When a sufferer is close to his past suffering, memory can bring a very vivid picture of those upsetting experiences. Small wonder that memory becomes accompanied by apprehension and a nagging dread that 'it' may return.

The writer said that he is almost cured. To be so near cure he has surely learned how to accept and so quieten some nervous symptoms. He can do this again. He should encourage himself with that thought, and instead of staying tensely on guard, trying to keep setback at bay, he should face the niggly fear and be prepared to let the symptoms come, full blast if necessary. If he does this, the niggly fear will gradually subside. The subsidence is quicker if he has an opportunity, not once but several times (even more than several), to pass through the return of symptoms successfully. Always, no-longer-mattering holds the key that brings future peace with no more niggling fear.

I said 'no more niggling fear'. However, the truth is that even when the return of symptoms no longer matters, carrying niggling fear can become a habit and can persist for some time. Once again, acceptance and letting time pass are joint healers.

THAT PERSISTENT INNER VOICE

There is a persistent inner voice that challenges the nervous person to think the worst; a little voice that says, 'Others can do it, others can recover, but not you!' A nervously ill person's mind can play strange tricks and he is too easily impressed by them. He doesn't understand that it is natural for an inner voice to complain as his does, while he is still so sensitized.

Recovery often follows similar patterns and one of these is the frequent development of a negative inner voice. Obstructive thoughts are normal, very human, in the circumstances. Their voice should be heard; let it have its way, it will take it, anyhow. Let it say what it wants to; let it bring plenty of fear but *watch it doing it*; while you have the courage to watch without letting it overpower you, you will gradually feel yourself becoming detached from its babbling.

FAINTING

Very few nervously ill people faint. From time to time, many 'feel faint', but few actually faint. This is because the faintness a nervously ill person experiences is so often self-induced and most sufferers, when they start to work themselves up for fear they will faint, usually manage to divert their attention from the fainting to finding an escape route. They are so used to defeating their feeling of faintness by flight, they always sit near a door, so that they can depart quickly if necessary.

But why do they feel faint in the first place? I'm not talking about the person who has been only 'picking at' his food and is possibly undernourished, anaemic. I speak of a nervously ill but adequately fed person. Such a person feels faint because he, in any feared situation, continuously gives himself little shocks by suggesting, 'What if I have to sit near the front? ... How much longer will I be able to sit through this? ... Will that man *never* stop talking? ... What if I do faint? ... I can feel it coming! ... What if I can't get out, and faint?' Shock after shock. Most people's nerves can stand this onslaught for a long time and the victim may feel only light-headed. As I said, the nervously ill person rarely faints.

The lesson to be learnt is that no nervously ill person need faint if he, or she, is prepared to do as I'm constantly advising – and that is, to not add second-fear. If you are in the situation where you fear fainting, let your body go loose (relax) to the best of your ability and be prepared to accept whatever feelings it brings without adding the extra shock of 'Oh, my goodness, what's going to happen now!'

It is strange how we keep our grip on ourselves by being prepared to release it. We never keep the right kind of grip by holding tensely on to ourselves, as so many wrongly believe. By abandoning ourselves to whatever our body may care to do, we release the tension that is fatiguing the nerves controlling our blood vessels, and they are able to contract normally and prevent blood pooling in our legs; we also relieve the stress that may sometimes activate the vagus nerve to slow the heart's beating. After a while we do not even feel faint.

So much of a nervously ill person's suffering is self-induced through ignorance and bewilderment. It is also induced by what he thinks is the hovering shadow of having some day, somehow, to face the ultimate.

No-one is quite sure what he means by this, but each is convinced that it is something terrible. The ULTIMATE – in other words, the worst that could possibly happen – is no more than a creation of fear and imagination working together – a bogyman that will disappear if the sufferer has the courage to say 'Boo!'

Some people do faint more readily than others, whether they are nervously ill or not; for example, soldiers on parade, who stand for hours in the same place. This kind of faintness can be corrected by moving one's body as much as the situation permits.

Please don't think, after reading this, that if you have to stand still anywhere that you must immediately begin to fidget. As it is, the nervously ill person who stands quite still for any length of time would be hard to find. Remember, no nervous person need faint because of his 'nerves' if he lets his body loosen and accepts whatever feelings it brings him, even the sensation of 'feeling faint'.

FEAR OF DYING

I could tell you that 'what can't be cured must be endured' and so it must, but how to endure a fear of death that may haunt for years – sometimes a lifetime – while yet being prepared to face death when it actually comes? That is the point.

Sudden death gives no time for its contemplation, so why should we fear it? It seems foolish to worry about something we would know nothing about, and yet, so many are afraid of sudden death. Many nervously ill people fear that, at the peak of their panic, they may collapse and die. They read about people who do die in a moment of extreme emotional stress and they see themselves doing the same.

During my experience as a doctor treating hundreds of nervously ill people, I have not known one to die during a panic spell. I suspect that the people we have read about who died this way already had a 'heart condition' and that the extra stress was the last straw. Nervously ill people have, as a rule, experienced so much panic that their heart has already shown them, again and again, how much it can endure; indeed, they often have very strong hearts. Trust your powers of adaptation. They will not fail you as readily as you may imagine.

While some people are concerned with sudden death, most are concerned with death that may come gradually, when they are old. Here again, I speak as a doctor. I have rarely attended a person actually dying who realized that he, or she, was dying. A few do, but very few. Nature blunts the edge of her sword; even during the years before our death nature helps us; our habits, our demands on life change. At 20, the weekend means activity – dinner and dance and tennis; at 70, we'd rather sit by the fire and read. Activity naturally slows down. If we are prepared to go along with nature as willingly as possible, she will make our death rather like our birth – while we will be the star performer, we will be unaware of the performance.

I don't say that there may not be suffering for many during those last months – even years – but here again, age dulls feeling to a certain extent; inevitability brings its own anaesthesia.

Creatures of adaptation that we are, we adapt even to the thought of death. Let me tell you about one old man. He needed an operation on his throat. The surgeon explained that if he had the operation his life could be prolonged by as much as three or four years. The man asked, 'How long will I live if I don't have the operation?' The surgeon replied, 'About six months.'

'Then', said the patient, 'I'll settle for six months, thank you. If I go into hospital I'll lose my lodgings and they're very hard to find these days!'

I remember looking at the man in amazement. The surgeon, elderly himself, showed no surprise. He turned and said to us – his group of students – 'The philosophy of old age!' Understanding this was beyond me. Today, I understand it well.

Youth and middle age are for active living and we should not rob it of any of its joy by dreading something that, when it comes, we may actually welcome, or at least, may be unaware of its approach. I remember a woman of 80 who had feared the thought of dying all her life. When the time came she said to me, 'I don't mind dying. I've seen everything and I've been everywhere and I'm very tired. Elsie's gone. Fred's gone. Funny, isn't it, I feel more part of them than I do of the people here. There's not much pleasure left now. What a silly I've been all these years worrying about dying. Now I want to go!' It is so often like that.

Another woman of 84 saw her grandchild, aged four, for the first time. She said, 'This has made living through the last few years worthwhile!' And yet to outsiders, including her family, she'd seemed happy enough during those last years. So when she did die her daughter always had the comforting thought, 'Mother didn't mind going, really!'

Have you ever thought that going through a surgical operation must be very like dying? As we're given the injection, we are asked to count; by the time we reach number seven, we're back in bed, with sister bending over us asking us if we feel all right? And yet three or four hours may have passed between 'seven' and the vision of sister. What happened to us during that time? Nothing we know about. Did those four hours worry us? No, they were as nothing. Surely death is not so very different? If you are religious and believe in life after death you have in-built comfort; if you have no such belief, remember that operation and comfort yourself with the thought, 'Why be afraid of something I will know nothing about?'

Therefore, however old you may be, live each day as it comes and always plan for the future. If, when you are 90, you need a new tea set, buy it. Don't think, 'I won't buy that. It's too late!' If you have only a little time to enjoy, enjoy it with what time you have, and enjoy it right up to the very last minute. The days that come when you aren't there won't worry you, because you won't be there to be worried!

Concern yourself only with the days you are alive and enjoy them to their full. Leave the rest to Nature, or to God, as you prefer, and never be bluffed into fearing death, however you imagine it may come.

THE FIRST PANIC

'The first time I panicked was out shopping in Exeter. I'd had a cup of tea in the store and had gone up to the powder room. I felt so panicky I asked to be taken home. That experience so upset me, I didn't go to Exeter for ages.

'I panicked again three weeks later. I was tense at the time, having been to the dentist a few days earlier; a set appointment always worries me. Just two days later came my granddaughter's christening. It was a lovely service in a delightful church and I enjoyed it very much. There was a buffet meal afterwards at a local hotel. I enjoyed watching the people looking after my mother (she was 85) and helping my 18-month-old granddaughter with her meal. I got chocolate on my hands and decided to wash them.

'I know the hotel well but the powder room is newly built and strange. It was empty when I got there. I can see now the connection between the panic in Exeter and the panic on this occasion. The trouble started when I locked the toilet door. I always find locking doors threatening. First comes the fear and then everything seems to recede. I know what I am and what I am doing but I seem to be in a dream, to have lost my identity. I remember at Exeter wondering if I was still alive. In the middle of all this, I remembered Dr Weekes saying, "Take no notice of strange feelings. Loosen and accept!"

'I washed my hands and they took ages to dry under the dryer. I looked in the mirror. I felt awful and I looked awful, and thought, "I'll do my hair and powder my nose and then go back." This I did. I then went back along the corridor to the dining room, sat down and carried on where I had left off. The feeling of panic had almost subsided.

'The next day I was very tired but I decided that I would not be put out by it this time although I kept remembering it.

'Doctor, had the feeling reached its peak or could it have got worse? Was it likely to have lasted any longer? If that was "it", I know I can cope with it again should it recur.'

To wish for reassurance that 'it' could grow no greater shows that this woman still fears panic and while she is afraid she harbours the seeds of further panic. For her, 'it' certainly could have got worse had she not coped the way she did. She must try not to rest secure in the feeling 'I can stand *that* much!' She must know that *she can face and go through panic however fiercely it may come*. She can have this comfort: even the fiercest flash has its limit! Only when she can pass through any flash the right way will she lose fear of both 'it' and the menacing shadow of 'perhaps!'.

Panic takes many strange forms and 'recession' is one of them. I talk about this in my book, *Peace from Nervous Suffering*, and have already mentioned it in this book. Recession is a feeling of thoughts going back, back, right to the very back of the head; frightening, because the sufferer wonders if he will ever come back to be himself again. Recession is no more than tension's screws clamping more tightly than usual – a feeling of being encased in one's own mind – identity lost! It is essential to recognize and not be bluffed by tension's strange tricks. The calmness that comes with the relaxation (even the slightest) that understanding brings (it came to this woman to some extent when she remembered my words and returned to her friends) helps to unclamp the clamp. There is nothing to fear.

This woman's next question was about going to Tavistock even though feeling unwell. She said, 'I now think I can cope with panic on travelling, but when I'm not well I can't decide whether it's just an excuse or should I make myself go?'

'Not well' is a vague expression. If she had influenza with a temperature, she certainly should not go – moderation in all things. However, while she wonders if she is making an excuse, she can't be very ill. So, if there is good reason to be at Tavistock, she should go – doubts and all.

If she decides not to go, accepting this negative decision (unless the thermometer says: stay!) will be very difficult. Most nervously ill people find accepting negative decisions difficult, especially if there is a shadow of doubt. For example, this woman would think, 'Perhaps I should have gone! Perhaps I'm being cowardly!'

True acceptance means accepting a negative decision once it is made. Swinging from 'Perhaps I should have!' to 'Perhaps I shouldn't!' is tiring and confusing and does nothing for confidence. Going to Tavistock to face an obligation there despite feeling 'lousy' is a great confidence booster. In my first book, I say, 'Wait on no mood.' The mood-waiter waits one heck of a long time!

So, off to Tavistock!

CHAPTER 4

❧

Journals to Patients 1975–82

During 1968–70, I sent quarterly journals of encouragement to approximately 1300 nervously ill people (mainly in the United Kingdom) who were using my book *Self Help for Your Nerves*, and my recordings* for recovery. These journals were published in my book, *Peace from Nervous Suffering*.

In 1971 I made a survey of approximately 500 of these people, which was published in the *British Medical Journal*, May 26, 1973.

During 1972–74 I continued sending quarterly journals which I condensed into a composite journal and published in my book, *Simple, Effective Treatment of Agoraphobia*.

During 1975–82 I sent one journal yearly – quarterly journals were no longer needed as so many people were recovering. These journals are published here.

A casual reader may query the repetition in these journals; however, the nervously fatigued, or nervously ill, person will recognize repetition as treatment. He wants the advice stressed

* For a full list of Dr Weekes' cassettes and recordings, and information on where to obtain them, see p. 425.

until he *feels* it, not only reads it. He needs the motivation feelings brings; repetition emphasizes and so encourages feeling.

The following journals were sent to approximately 2000 nervously ill people, mainly agoraphobic, in the United Kingdom, the United States of America, Canada, Australia and Africa during 1975–82.

MAY 1975

Willingly

Once more I write to you from Australia. Sometimes I must leave England or the United States to return to my family out here. However, I think of you and often wonder about your progress. I have said so much in books, tapes, journals, that it will be difficult for you not to know, almost by heart, what I want you to do and how to do it. And yet there may be many of you who still need encouragement and guidance.

It is possible to reduce all my messages to a few simple words. Actually, my teaching can be reduced to one word. If you asked me what, of all I have taught you, you should remember, I would say: remember to try to always act WILLINGLY. Willingly face the day, willingly take what comes and especially willingly (as willingly as you can manage, to begin with) accept the symptoms you dislike so much. Remember that word willingly, willingly, WILLINGLY. However, don't try to let willingly work for you until you have been assured by your doctor that your symptoms are caused by 'nerves'.

Although I have talked to you about almost every aspect of your nervous illness, I have not yet discussed those years 'lost' in illness. During your illness you have naturally concentrated so much on yourself that you have not fully lived in the outside world (that is putting it mildly for some of you) so that those years seem lost; as if there is a no-man's land between you – as you are now – and that earlier, well you.

Actually, you've learned a great deal during those apparently lost years. You've learned to be compassionate, how to understand and possibly help others and how to appreciate simple things. It may seem as if your normal life came to an abrupt end when you first became ill, and that there is an unbridgeable gap between then and now. It seems unbridgeable because you are looking back and are trying to build a bridge *behind* you to link up with today. The bridge can be built only by going quietly forward until the feeling of normality, which recovery gradually brings, builds it. Then you find yourself automatically linking up with the old you.

I appreciate that some of you are still battling, and haven't made the progress you think you should have made. This is most probably because you haven't practised the way I've taught you, or the conditions in which you are trying to recover have been especially discouraging, or you may have been physically ill. I know some of you have been physically ill and have carried on in spite of this. This is true courage.

If you carry out my teaching the right way in spite of failures in the past, you will recover; so, however disappointed or discouraged you may be, start practising again WILLINGLY. I especially want to encourage those who have done well, who even thought they were over the final hurdle, perhaps even recovered, and who in spite of this are now in a setback. This can be almost devastatingly disappointing. However, nothing you have learned has been lost, so don't whip yourself because you think you have slipped from the right path after so much success, and don't exhaust yourself wondering how it could have happened to you! You may even be the mainstay of a special group of nervously ill people and view your setback as a special calamity. Actually it will help you revise your knowledge of nervous suffering and of how to come out of it. It may even help you to be more patient with those others who seem stuck in a rut in their illness. Being obliged to come through setback yet again may even humble you and we're all better for a touch of humbling now and then.

So, I want to encourage those discouraged to start once more. I think of you struggling away in those far lands. You are such brave people. Don't drop out of the recovery race however many your past failures may be. Failure counts only if you let it.

JANUARY 1976

Defusing the Bomb

It hardly seems fair that I should be talking to you in bright sunshine while so many of you are in the cold and rain. However, you did have a good summer last year didn't you?

In this letter I will talk about *defusing the bomb*.

Some nervously ill people think they are accepting by 'learning to live with' their illness. (Even some doctors say, 'You'll have to learn to live with this!') That is, some people are prepared to compromise and live with some aspect of their illness without making an effort to rid themselves permanently of all of it. They are resigned to some defeat. This is not the *right* kind of acceptance. I want you to learn how to cope with your illness until you are free of all of it – no compromise. I don't want those who are agoraphobic to resign themselves permanently to not go here, not go there, not travel in this or that.

The acceptance I teach means going forward, doing the things dreaded and doing them with utter acceptance of whatever nervous symptoms, sensations, experiences may come while doing them. It means accepting even revulsion against the thought of doing and still doing: but DOING the right way (you remember? – the deep breath, the letting go and the marching forward?). Yesterday I showed a woman how she was agitating herself by withdrawing from the thought of the situation she feared. For her it was flying from Sydney to Melbourne two days later, and she hardly knew how she would live through those two days.

I explained it was as if she had a lemon in her tummy which she squeezed every time she thought of that menacing journey, and that the more she squeezed the more agitated she became because the more stress hormone she produced. I said, 'Take your hand off that lemon. Don't keep squeezing it!' She had already learnt how to cope with panic after 40 years of misery but did not appreciate that she should cope with agitation the same way. It was the feeling of agitation, of restlessness, that upset her now.

I taught her to go forward into the agitation; to let herself *be agitated*; to stop withdrawing in apprehension from it, to even try relaxing toward it. In other words, to stop continually squeezing that lemon.

She managed the journey home and telephoned today. She said that what helped her most was the thought, 'Hands off that lemon!'

If you are like this, when you go forward into your fears, even into agitation, you gradually DEFUSE THE BOMB. Every time you come out of setback, you have defused it a little more; every time you practise the right way, you defuse it still further. Some day, when you do something daring, like visiting a distant town or riding on your own in a bus or train, you will find that even though you expect to panic, *panic does not come*. Your practice at acceptance has finally taken the power out of panic, the fuse out of the bomb. This doesn't mean that you will never panic again. Far from it. That old demon will certainly appear again; but once the bomb has been defused, panic loses its power to bluff you. There may be short bursts (even a long one!), but you are able to pass through these with understanding and confidence.

Also, instead of being overwhelmed and discouraged by setback, I want you to understand that to be able to be in a setback means that you must have previously made progress. Be glad of that and accept the setback as part of recovery and quietly go on. As I said, every time you come through setback you defuse the bomb still further. It all adds up, so don't waste a good setback lamenting about it. Use it for further defusing. Make the most of it.

I have mentioned the strange tricks that fatigue can play. There is that strange ability to do things well one day, and yet, the next day, be unable to even contemplate doing them. We make the mistake of judging ourselves while we are fatigued, without recognizing our incompetence as fatigue.

I'm still impressed by the fatigued nervously ill person's inability to quickly change a point of view. On the other hand, I am intrigued by his ability to do this if he approaches the change gradually, with quiet but relaxed determination. Gradually is the key word. All comes gradually. Set your goal and float toward it. You can't strenuously argue yourself better. If you try, you will not stop arguing. Getting better is a job for time and continued acceptance (or repeated trial at acceptance!).

Fatigue also underlies much depression, especially the fatigue of repeatedly doing uninteresting things. But even here, if work is done willingly and spirits are not being continually drained, a natural resilience helps to carry one above mundane tasks. By willingly I mean to even willingly carry the 'heart of lead', the 'horse's hoof' in the tummy, to work with this aching heaviness and not try agitatedly to find something to do to distract and help lose it. To go forward in depression with willing acceptance will work a miracle. This teaching is based on physiological laws which have always worked and always will. Trust them.

For those of you who have worked and progressed well, my thanks and congratulations. For those still struggling, don't lose heart. Have some more shots at defusing the bomb. But make sure you understand clearly what I have taught you.

JULY 1976

The Front Line of Battle

When I heard that the temperature in Britain was 90°, I wished I had taught you more about the similarity between some of the symptoms of nervous illness and those felt during very hot weather: those flushes that seem almost like mini-panics, the pounding heart, the feeling of fullness in the face, the sweating, fatigue and so on.

So, don't be discouraged during the heat by any symptoms resembling nervous symptoms: always remember that these are the usual symptoms that can come with stress, and a very hot day can be stressful; so please don't be tricked into thinking that they mean the return of your illness.

Some of you want so badly to lose your symptoms, you keep yourselves in an almost constant state of anxiety about it, and because of the stress anxiety brings, the symptoms persist. Can you understand this? You are like a dog with a can tied to its tail, round and round he goes, trying to get rid of it. You go round in a cycle, *anxiously* trying to be rid of the symptoms of anxiety that of course then chase you!

So I want to give a special prescription to those who are tired of revolving in that cycle. First: try to be less anxious about the symptoms. If you can manage only a little less anxiety, there will be less stress and the symptoms, because of this, must calm a little. Second: play my cassettes* as often as you can manage. Make this effort. Some of the cassettes are long, so don't necessarily play the entire cassette at one sitting. Now – and here comes the important pat of this prescription – at this stage you need only listen. You need not even try to go out and practise what I teach you. JUST LISTEN, but again and again.

After you have spent a week or more listening, you will absorb more of my teaching than you realize and one day, when out, if you have one of your crippling 'spells', you will find that you have an in-built little voice that supports and tells you what to do. What is more, you will find yourself automatically doing it. So, those of you who are tired and discouraged and feel like giving up, GIVE UP, but play the cassettes and listen. You will be surprised at the result.

This morning a woman reminded me of an aspect of recovery from nervous illness that I can never emphasize too much. It is the strangeness, especially during the early stages. This woman, who had been complaining of feeling unreal, said that during the previous weekend, as soon as she started practising its acceptance, the feeling of unreality had come more vividly than ever, and more often than before. She was now confused and worried, because she was sure she had done everything I had advised. She said she had accepted the feeling, had not tried to puzzle out what it meant, and not even tried to get rid of it or run away from it. She had even been prepared to work with it there. Yet, it stayed. She couldn't understand this.

* For a full list of Dr Weekes' cassettes and recordings, and information on where to obtain them, see p. 425.

This woman had not done *everything* that I had advised her. She had forgotten that I had warned her in my books that this very experience could occur and is what deters so many people from trying to recover on their own without any outside help. As soon as they begin to question if they are working the right way or not, they fall into the trap of being at first bewildered and then despairing. They feel bereft; they think even my teaching has failed them: there is no hand to grasp.

I reminded her that in my book I wrote that in the beginning, when a sufferer first practises what I teach, he is deliberately putting himself in the front line of battle, putting his head on the block. It has to be like this, because instead of pushing a disliked feeling aside (and this sometimes works for a while), he faces it, may even go looking for it. Being ready to practise coping with what is feared often means concentrating on it. This woman's decision to try to cope with the feeling of unreality that weekend so alerted her to it, that it became a highlight of the weekend.

Although she was comforted by this explanation, I expected her to have a gruelling week; however if she continued as I had taught her – with willing acceptance of the feeling – it would gradually become less and less important until it would hardly ruffle her.

Everything comes back to willing acceptance. Sometimes I write the words 'Willing acceptance' on a prescription form for a patient. Some print it in large letters on a card which they hang in a prominent place in their home – usually over the kitchen sink.

Will you try once more to do as I teach you? If it's only to play the cassettes and listen. I send you all my encouragement.

OCTOBER 1997

A Miracle From Within

If only I could gather you all together and really drive the message home that recovery lies in your understanding of acceptance and practising it and not in expecting an outside miracle. I did speak to some of you in London this year, and to others in Liverpool.

Recently I helped a woman through a period of nervous 'exhaustion' when she thought she'd reached the end of her tether and couldn't go one step further. She had been doing very well, and had even held down a job, but now she was at the stage where she could hardly find the energy to take the car out of the garage to take her little girl to school. Earlier in the month she had had a 'queer turn' while out, and this is why she had worked herself up into a proper state about driving into town. She was at the stage of thinking, 'I'll never go near that place again!'

So, we started off from taws – exhaustion, panic, influenza, family illness and complete (or so she thought) lack of confidence, with added unwillingness to go on with the struggle. But gradually, by encouraging her to go out while she was so 'done', she came to see that she could still function even in those 'terrible' moments. By working at those times, she gradually built a little platform of confidence from which to go into town, drive her daughter to school and even visit her sick relative in hospital.

On one occasion I spoke harshly to her. I have rarely done this to any patient. I was so exasperated, because I had spoken to her so often, and she knew so well what she had to do to recover, but was making no effort. I wanted to shake her out of herself and I succeeded. Although she is still very, very tired and upset by a recent death in the family and has *another* cold, she says she knows she's on the right road again. She has glimpsed recovery once more, because she no longer baulks at doing things when she 'doesn't feel like it'. She no longer waits until she feels better. She has found the eye of the hurricane.

Sailors say that in the middle of a hurricane there is a place of peace, which they call the eye. To find it the ship must first pass through the storm. This woman had faced and passed through while the storm raged, and although her symptoms did not disappear, she felt the peace of achievement and the beginning of being freed from her chains. She understood that with the new inner peace she now had, the symptoms would gradually calm.

This letter is to encourage you to find the eye of your hurricane; so, onward little ship into the storm, into the eye of the hurricane, but willingly with acceptance.

OCTOBER 1978

Clearing Away the Mists

Gauging the stage of your progress is difficult, so please forgive me if the following talk does not apply to you. However, there is surely some help in it for everyone. I am writing this in London. We are having an Indian summer and I'm not making the most of it because I've joined the band of the many who trip on a London pavement. I've sprained my foot. What a waste of such lovely weather!

In a letter recently, a woman wrote, 'Nobody can convince me that I won't go berserk, collapse, if I find myself in a situation I can't handle and when I'm a long way from home. How could I cope if I felt I couldn't stand another minute of it and there was no way to escape? Perhaps you could elaborate on this in some future article?'

In other words she longs for some cure outside herself that will rid her of her fear. She hasn't accepted yet that riddance must come from her. It would help her if she could see clearly just what would happen if she found herself in such a situation; now she sees it as if through a haze. Two factors are to be considered here. First, how can she stop the intensity of her panic building up and second, if she can't, what will happen then? She must understand that only she encourages her glands to keep secreting the chemicals that increase panic. I'm not talking about that flash, that lightning flash, of first-fear that seems to come automatically to a sensitized person in a frightening, or even only slightly frightening, situation; for example, a mere cold blast of wind! No-one, let alone a sensitized person, can immediately control that flash and I never ask them to. But this first, apparent, automatic flash, comes as one single flash. And always passes. *The panic that continues flashing must be added by the sufferer himself to that first flash.* And it is so very easy to add panic to panic, when sensitization triggers panic so easily.

Naturally panic that comes so easily bewilders the sufferer and she (here it is a woman) makes the mistake of thinking that it can, of its own accord, grow beyond her control. She does not understand clearly that panic can build up only if she builds it up. By doing as I have taught her so often by taking a deep breath, letting it out slowly, and letting her body slump – whether sitting or standing – and then being willing to let the panic flash, the panic will gradually decrease and there will never be a 'build up'.

So if that woman takes a journey in any vehicle she cannot stop at will, she should start the journey knowing that she will probably panic – fear of it will bring it – but also knowing that if she is prepared to sit and let the panic sweep through her *as willingly as she can manage*, THE PANIC WILL NOT MOUNT. But she must *stay* willing. So many manage to be willing at first, but if panic strikes again too soon after the first flash, they too easily forget willingness and start withdrawing in desperation and fear. Stopping panic mounting is in everybody's hands by not adding FEAR OF THE PANIC.

I know this sounds simple. It's not simple and I don't underestimate the strength of her panic, but she can do it and so can you.

The second part of the experience: suppose she does add panic to panic and the panic mounts, what then? Can there be a crisis so great that she can 'go berserk' or 'collapse'? There can't. Any movement she makes, no matter what, will thwart any crisis. For example, if she is in a train and gets up in panic and walks out into the corridor, the very getting up and walking defeats the peak of panic so that the moment of crises passes. Any diversion will blunt the peak of panic. This is a physiological fact. There is no such thing as a continuous crisis. The word 'crisis' means a turning point, a peak followed by a falling away. Even if that panicking woman only listens to the man opposite rustling his newspaper, some of her tension goes into listening and so the peak of that wave of panic passes. No peak goes on peaking continuously at the same level. Peaks always fall away on the other side.

She says she fears she may 'go berserk'. What does she mean by going berserk? I think she vaguely sees herself running away somewhere, arms waving, even crying out. But that's only hysteria and with the first burst she'd be so overcome by finding herself in the limelight, the hysteria would fizzle out like a damp firecracker. Such a person is always self-conscious and if there is one thing a self-conscious person does not do, it's to cry out.

But suppose she breaks all records and does cry out; what then? At the first cry she'd be so overcome with shame, she'd slink back into her seat and I doubt if she'd have enough strength to panic again on that journey. She is letting the possibility of feeling humiliated before other people – people she'd probably never see again – spoil her life. Wouldn't it be better for her to face the worst bravely and so free herself from her self-created prison? And incidentally, a 'worst' that is only part of her imagination. What chains her misty vision is creating!

Also, what does she mean by 'collapse'? She doesn't understand 'collapse' clearly either, or she wouldn't use the word. To truly collapse – medically speaking – one's blood pressure must fall dramatically. In a panic, blood pressure usually goes up not down, so how could she collapse? And yet at the moment of peak-panic, some people complain that they feel light-headed or muzzy, as if they are going to collapse. One woman referred to her 'blackouts', but when questioned critically, she admitted that she never lost consciousness, only felt that she might. I have been called out to visit a patient, whom relatives described as 'collapsed', only to have her laughing after a few minutes talk.

If the woman who wrote that letter did work herself up so that she felt light-headed, muzzy, and then slumped on to the floor with fright and weakness, someone would always help her to her feet again and she'd always find a good excuse to explain the 'collapse'.

So what? So what? I wish you would ask yourselves that question. *The courage to go out and face any crisis, whatever it may be, is enough to dampen it.* Can you see that? You are holding only a firecracker (even though it may be a double-bunger!) in your hand and letting that spoil your life!

At a Canadian hospital, a doctor had biro pens stamped with a quote from one of my books, 'Recovery lies in the places and experiences you avoid'. Never run away from such places or experiences. They are your salvation because recovery truly lies in them.

So, clear away the mists. Understand that the controls are in your hands and that you work those controls by releasing them. Understand that even if you cling on and fail to release them and let panic mount and mount, it can only, in the end, spend itself. A wave that breaks on the beach, however big, must always recede. Let no vaguely imagined crisis spoil your life.

OCTOBER 1979

Keep Trucking

Once again I greet you and once again I have the problem of not knowing how much you personally need this letter and how much you want simply to keep in touch. As those who need help must be served first I will write as if you, the reader of this letter, are one of them. Many of you are making good progress, and may not want to be reminded of the details of your illness and yet, for the sake of others I must give details.

As I have said so often, the most upsetting symptom of sensitized nerves is the intensity of the body's reaction to the slightest anxious thought, and the consequent self-bombardment by fear of this reaction, even to the extent of the sufferer thinking that he, or she, is going mad.

Pcace and rest. How they are longed for and how unattainable they seem. I'm saddened by the number of exhausted people who have no-one to turn to for help. I ask, 'Isn't there *some* relative or friend with whom you can stay, if only for a little while? Someone who will keep you company during the day and give you a change from loneliness and work?' The answer is so often, 'No-one!' or, 'Only Mum and she doesn't understand.

Essential Help for your Nerves

Anyhow I've worn her out!' One woman when telephoning me had to ring off if she heard her husband coming; he was so fed up with her illness. Too often, the way out must be found alone.

Peace lies in finding a satisfactory way of looking at any problem that is helping to keep the sufferer ill; in finding a route to follow (as I have been teaching you) and then, in 'keepin' truckin''. Indecision and the bewilderment it brings debilitate, especially if the sufferer is constantly changing his mind and is reacting too intensely to each change. If you suffer this way and understand the effects of sensitization and fatigue and see that it is not necessarily the situation that is causing your present state as much as your too severe reaction to it – especially your reaction to the anxieties, fears, associated with it – then, if you can do this, you are on the road to recovery. I know acceptance is very difficult if you live under constant tension at home or at work; but when you do accept (and everybody has the power to do this) your nervous reactions will gradually lessen, fatigue lift, and what has seemed impossible for so long gradually becomes possible.

But don't try to push yourself to show that you 'can do it!' Take short rests if necessary. Utter tiredness may be 'only nerves' but it feels like utter tiredness just the same. Unfortunately, sleeping during the day can seem more like a nightmare than rest. The fatigued person can wake with such a start (we call this the 'startles') that his heart may race and he may feel 'flat', depressed, for some hours afterwards. If you wake this way, don't think you are uniquely or especially ill. Your body is following an expected pattern which is part of sensitization.

As I have mentioned again and again, having someone with whom to discuss your problem helps tremendously, especially someone who will encourage you. Helpful discussion releases tension, unties the knotted chest, the clamped scalp, the tight throat. It helps lift the bag of concrete from the heart. However, only too often the sufferer talks indiscriminately to too many people and some acquaintances are not only unhelpful but have the knack of saying the wrong thing, which sets the sufferer off on another track of misery.

Grotesque, frightening thoughts are not unusual in debilitated people who have no defence against their own imagination – especially fearful imagination. Rest and peace (those beautiful experiences) will come if the sufferer understands and accepts depletion and knows that no devil has him in his power; if he understands that all is caused by sensitization, fatigue and memory playing their tricks. (But what a devil they can seem! I was too quick saying there was no devil!)

Tranquillizers are sometimes essential, but a wise doctor's direction is necessary.

Change in the pattern of everyday living can act like a mild shock, arresting the sufferer's constant thinking about himself and how he feels. It helps him to suddenly see himself 'from the outside', to feel on top of his illness as if detached from it; this enables him to get it into proportion. Simply leaving the house and walking outside can lift the grey veil of mental fatigue a little. If only for a short time. To be able to get away from the house for a month or more is a rare luxury. Most people must stay and recover in the old tracks at home. Recovery is still possible here, but it may take longer.

If you suffer this way, try to see your illness as nervous fatigue from which you will recover if you are willing to accept the strange feelings and sensations, and try to let time pass while waiting for recovery, especially if you are willing to pass through those flash moments when symptoms return so vividly and make you think, all too readily, that you never will be free of them, will never recover.

Let them come, those strange flashes, let all the strange feelings flash back. Even let the stomach churn. Release your tense hold on them and 'keep truckin' '. But keep trucking willingly, without tensely fighting. And don't keep trying 'to get rid of them'. No-one can get rid of 'them' quickly. Only if you work as willingly as you can *with the feelings there*, will you gradually be rid of them.

This advice also applies to depressed people. Depression is a chemical disturbance; this is why anti-depressants sometimes help. If you are depressed and understand that it is a chemical disturbance and try not to be depressed because you are depressed, your batteries will gradually be recharged; the chemical imbalance will be remedied and depression will lift. So, be prepared to do things without continually watching to see if you are enjoying doing them. You couldn't suddenly switch from depression to enjoyment, except perhaps for an occasional quick flash.

Also, the last thing you may want to do is to mix with people. It can be almost painful to force your mind to concentrate on what others are saying, and as for sharing their enthusiasm over some everyday happening ...! But *you should mix with people*, however painful, and try not to pity yourself too much in the meantime. Try not to gauge your progress by the day, even by the week. Keep trucking and one morning you will wake without the lump of lead in your stomach, without the rattling heart, and gradually life will be worth living again.

I know this letter applies to only some of you. I apologize to the others. To all of you I send my compassionate understanding and best wishes.

Breaking Through the Barrier

Once again I send you my encouragement while you make that steep climb up the slippery slope. Recovery is such a slippery business, that I bring you special messages. Some of you may not understand what I'm talking about, but hundreds will and these may still need a steadying hand.

Recovery can be slow because emotions, felt as intensely as a sensitized person can feel them, can bring some off-putting shocks. The word 'shock' may surprise you; however, to the sensitized person a thought or an experience, that brings the slightest anxiety or surprise, can feel like a physical shock.

For example, as I have mentioned before, a nervously ill person who stays indoors most of the time may be so accustomed to the subdued light inside the house that simply opening the front door to venture out into the bright light can bring such a physical jolt that the would-be adventurer may quickly retreat indoors, defeated.

Again, while recovering, those moments of having a peaceful body may feel so strange, the sudden realization that one's body is at peace may shock and of course when this happens back come the old fears and bewilderment – plenty of bewilderment. Certainly bewilderment, because where does one go from there? If feeling at peace brings shock, where *does* one go from there?

Even the thought of full recovery may be daunting, even slightly shocking. The sufferer feels that the vitality demanded by recovery seems beyond his reach. He would almost rather stay ill. He feels he will never be able to make the effort to walk briskly, laugh freely, talk unselfconsciously. What a mountain to climb, especially when even a peaceful body seems strange. Again, there is recoil in shock.

He asks himself, 'How can I, how does anyone, break through such a barrier?' To break through, he *must let the moment of shock pass*; he must pass through, relax through, to the best of his ability, that flash-moment of fear and despair, and continue with the job on hand. HE MUST PASS THROUGH THAT FRONT DOOR INTO THE BRIGHT LIGHT. Always onward, onward.

With practice at passing through each blow, helped by an understanding that reactions are so severe because of sensitized response, the habit of being baulked is gradually replaced by the ability to pass (float, relax, melt) onward, through. When this happens, the shocks come more and more lightly until they NO LONGER MATTER. Finally, they are only a flickering memory and the barrier is gone.

The way is always onward, through, but there must be no grim fighting. Relaxed acceptance (as much as you can muster) of all obstacles, shocks, is the way through. This takes time, time, and much courage, patience, perseverance and picking oneself up from the depths of despair again and again, especially at first, when each blow seems to fall as forcefully as the last, sometimes even more forcefully. But then one day, as I said, comes that wonderful feeling that the shocks no longer matter. Not-mattering is usually fleeting at first – here one moment, gone the next. However, as the blows begin to soften, the former victim begins to feel an inner strength and a feeling that *he* is in charge of the situation at last. He no longer feels buffeted by some strange outside force working within himself. There is no outside force. There are only nerves responding to the stress born of fear, despair and a body's consequent fatigue. Fatigue can make the way seem so especially difficult. Acceptance and understanding gradually lift even fatigue.

I have not forgotten the shocks memory can bring. These are myriad. There are a few people who recover on waves of success, elation. The great majority, however, drag memory and its shocks along with them.

So, practise acceptance and always moving onward through all shocks until finally that wonderful moment of not-mattering is permanent. This is how recovery works. Shocks do not disappear by magic. They finally cease coming because THEY EVENTUALLY NO LONGER SHOCK.

Onward, onward, onward, accepting all, however shakily sometimes. Courage, each of you. You have my thoughts, my understanding and great sympathy as always.

JULY 1982

Where To From Here?

Some of you, who have been practising my teaching for some months and have been successful in moving about your own town – indeed may have achieved much in this way – may now be wondering, 'Where do I go from here?' So many have asked me this.

Many of you will remember how happy you were when you made the corner shop, the successful bus ride, the visit to the hairdressers. That was achievement. Sometimes it brought elation and relatives and friends, seeing the improvement, may have encouraged you. That was fine.

Your thoughts may now be, 'Perhaps if I were to go much further afield – somewhere really challenging – I would be satisfied?' But where? There is so little opportunity in ordinary life to go further afield. There's little encouragement to take a long journey to a place you don't know – perhaps just a name on a map, or on the front of a bus – simply to see if 'you can do it'.

If you were suddenly *obliged* to go to a distant town *that* would be different. There's a real push behind 'having to go' and a real push is a wonderful starter. If only the average daily life held more pushes. But it doesn't.

So, with travelling around the home town conquered, many people begin to worry, because they think they'll never be cured unless they at least have a go at some distant prospect, something that gives them a few cold shivers to contemplate. They don't realize that they could make that heroic effort, that distant journey, successfully and still have that gnawing, unsatisfied feeling deep within themselves of not having achieved enough.

If you are like this, what are you going to do about it? Let me assure you that if you are prepared to continue willingly with your apparently (or, at least, so it seems to you) humdrum living without trying to conquer further fields to convince yourself that you can get there, *you will be recovering all the time.*

Recovery, without your knowledge, is being cemented at your home-base by your simply doing the things that come fairly comfortably and perhaps without too much conscious effort on your part. You may be surprised to find that if making some unusually long journey – perhaps an hour or two away from home – is necessary, although you may have plenty of misgivings when you think about it and especially when you start off, all those months of successful (even if only sometimes fairly successful) ordinary living add up and you will make the journey more easily than you thought possible. Even while you think you are achieving little, you are achieving much. And that is exactly where you go next – to the shops, the school meeting, the hairdresser, and not in your dreams to Land's End or over the Brooklyn Bridge.

You see, two or three long journeys, although exciting and, if successful, very encouraging, can also disappoint because such efforts can only be spasmodic and there is no certainty about spasmodic effort. The only certainty lies within yourself and how you tackle the moments of panic *right on your doorstep*. That is, by seeing panic through until it matters less and less, by going to the other side of panic and finding peace there as I have taught so often. *Going to distant places is not necessary for your recovery*.

While you are coping with yourself in your own home town, you are, at the same time, coping with a distant journey. But you won't be successful in this if you move freely around your own town simply because you have 'become used to' doing it. There is no real, permanent peace, in getting-used-to. You must have the inner knowledge of going through panic the right way. Only in this way can confidence to face distant journeys be slowly, subconsciously built. Confidence cannot be built successfully unless the foundation is right. If you have come a certain distance by working the right way and are wondering where you go from there, and if you are distressed because nothing far afield offers itself, don't think you won't progress unless you find such a field. You will be getting better all the time if you settle contentedly with what is available at home, providing you are tackling it the right way.

I'll explain again what I mean by recovery. Even when you can do things you previously could not do, memory may sometimes encourage that old demon, panic, to rattle his chains. However, the rattling gradually grows less and less as you cope with it the right way, until it finally fades and is only a thought without too much upsetting bodily reaction. Memory may bring a slight shiver of apprehension (for months, perhaps for years) but what the heck! We can't anaesthetize memory.

I don't want to discourage anyone who has his, or her, heart set on taking a long journey. If you feel like this you have all my encouragement. So on with your spurs and call for your horse. You'll make it. Remember, you take your cure with you if you loosen and accept.

I am really writing this for the people who have no opportunity to call for a horse. I want to assure them that if they cope with what is at hand the right way, they are coping with that distant journey at the same time. I send you all my encouragement, my thoughts.

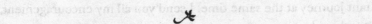

CHAPTER 5

More Bewilderments Cleared

COPING WITH A NEIGHBOUR

'How does one cope when out and the neighbour stops to talk and you feel you are going to collapse, or something dreadful is going to happen? What can I do instead of making the usual excuses of, "I must go. I've left the kettle on!" or, "I'm waiting for a phone call!" At home and in the house, I can let go and flop into the chair, but in the street this is impossible. The neighbour may be thinking, "She's not listening!"

'This makes me dread going out; yet I still go, because I know we have to go into the situations we fear. You say so. You see, I often feel queer before I go out – with light-headedness, stiff legs and weakness, yet I know I haven't been anticipating this and once outside, how unreal and strange I feel! Then, if anyone stops me, I've had it!

'I'm the same in the library, if I'm waiting to be served with people behind me. I can't say, "Just a minute while I try to relax!" I think you understand what I mean. It's so bewildering and makes me feel such a failure, especially when I come home to an empty house with no-one to talk to or to encourage me.

'Also, I'm terribly agitated if anyone visits and I don't know them very well. That's a nightmare. The young couple next door asked me in for coffee one day and a few days later I passed a cup of tea over to them. I said I couldn't go in because I was expecting Bill. I couldn't face the agitation of visiting, although they know I'm not very well.'

When you are stopped by a neighbour think to yourself, 'Float, just float, float, float! Don't fight!' Take a deep breath, let it out slowly and at the same time, let your body 'flop'. Your head may feel light, but it won't leave your shoulders! The stiff legs will hold you. These feelings are only tension working its old tricks. You can talk however tense and strange you feel. Your face won't crack if you smile.

If you can't follow every word your neighbour says, say you've got wax in your ears. What the heck! But don't run away to answer that phantom phone. See the talk through as WILLINGLY as you can manage. You'll be surprised what a miracle that old WILLINGLY will work. It begins by stopping that agitated searching for a way to escape.

You don't have to obviously sag or flop (although you probably could do both without the neighbour noticing). It's enough to think, 'Float!' and imagine yourself floating, to feel release of some tension.

When you stand in the queue at the library, once again think, 'Float, float, float!'

Visiting is always difficult for a nervously ill person. Here is a simple exercise you can do while visiting or being visited: surreptitiously clench one hand as tightly as you can and hold it clenched for about half a minute. When you unclench you will feel some relaxation. I doubt if your companions will be aware of the clenching. The release that follows clenching a hand can also relax tummy muscles.

You haven't been practising the right way, have you? Are those neighbours in, now? How about putting the kettle on?

IS DEPRESSION INHERITED?

In my opinion, depression may not be inherited as much as caused by environment. The mood of one member of a family can be too easily flattened by the depressed attitude of another member. For example, if on waking one is greeted by a cheerful mother, one is much more likely to step out of bed feeling that it's good to be alive, than if wakened by a depressed voice that lets one know that life's not worth much anyhow, so why bother?

Also if several members of the family suffer with depression, other members can too easily become afraid that they too will eventually suffer from it. A sure way to become depressed is to be constantly frightened; fear exhausts and depression is so often an expression of emotional exhaustion.

So if there is more than one member of your family suffering from depression, don't immediately think that you too must inevitably suffer from it. Don't fall into that trap.

TIMING

I first became aware of the importance of timing, while lecturing. I was rushing ahead trying to cram two hours into one. I wanted so earnestly to get the whole message across; I galloped. Suddenly I noticed a restlessness amongst the audience. I stopped; realized I was going too quickly, took a deep breath and continued slowly. By rushing I had been confusing them. Better, I thought to make six points clearly than garble a dozen. The fidgeting stopped. What's more I fitted in all the points and my pulse rate settled down.

We can develop our own tranquillization. Some simple kind of meditation in the morning and the afternoon will help to slow down the express train. There is no need to practise a form of meditation with a fancy name; I have my own simple form. For example, I sit quietly, close my eyes and with as little thought as possible, listen to outside noises. I used to do this in the middle of a busy surgery when it was impossible for me to take any other kind of rest. After a few minutes of listening quietly, I felt refreshed and my pace slowed down.

HOW TO RECOGNIZE THE BEGINNING OF DEPLETION

A woman wrote: 'I have just come through a crisis in my illness. I was greatly helped by your tape on Fatigue and realized that I need not feel guilty about my depression and weariness. Sometimes I think that we blame ourselves too much and all that is happening is that our mind is protesting and begging us to let go and, as you say, "let it all come". How can we learn to recognize the beginning of depletion? And after we have lived through depletion, how can we avoid it in the future, before it wears us down once more?'

Some of the early symptoms of depletion are: difficulty in concentrating, in deciding, in remembering; lessened interest, muzzy head, and irritability (too easily aroused emotions). At times there may be a flash of interest but it soon dies – too much effort! Acting on an idea is difficult.

However, one must remember that before depletion there must be much stress. Depletion does not follow physical work. It depends on glandular exhaustion, and physical work does not exhaust glands – only stress or disease can do that.

Living always on guard against depletion means being unnecessarily tense and this would soon invite fatigue, the forerunner of depletion. Better to arrange one's life sensibly within one's capacity and then forget about 'guarding against depletion'; at the same time remembering that how much one does is not as important as how one does it. If you are the kind of person who rushes through 'jobs to be done', practise timing. When you forget and do rush (as we all do at times) at least don't fret because you are rushing.

It's the anxiety added to fatigue that prolongs fatigue. Fatigue, even emotional and mental fatigue, will heal if we don't interfere by becoming anxious about it.

Often we get more relaxation by changing our work than by stopping working. Working with one's hands is a restful change for those who work constantly with their brain. The housewife may groan when she reads this because relaxation for her would be to forget that she had hands. For relaxation, she can lower her standards; if the beds aren't made on time, or even aren't made at all, so what!

TALKING TO OTHERS ABOUT FRIGHTENING THOUGHTS

Some ask if talking to others about their frightening thoughts is 'not accepting'.

Putting thoughts into words so often robs them of importance – they can suddenly seem silly. So talking about frightening thoughts to a *suitable confidant* can be good therapy. The confidant should be one who realizes the unimportance of the thoughts (although they may sound blood curdling!) and who doesn't withdraw in shock and say, 'You'll have to be careful, Willy, you could be going silly!' Not that kind of confidant.

During early stages in nervous illness, comforting words from others can sometimes break tension quicker than one's own anxious, desperate effort at self-comfort.

One woman found relief by saying to a particular friend, 'Please, Jean, repeat what I say to you.' Just hearing her own words coming from another's lips (even from someone who did not quite understand the meaning of the words) had more impact than saying them herself.

Hearing wise advice from cassettes* can help those who have no confidant.

BATTENING DOWN A VIVID IMAGINATION

'How can I batten down a vivid imagination?'

Don't try to. Give it full reign, but remember that it is only imagination. It is not a question of dampening a vivid imagination to gain peace, but of robbing imagination of its power to frighten. As one man put it, 'Recovery begins when the stupidities no longer matter.' One's imagination can certainly bring stupidities. Better to accept stupidities than try to batten imagination down!

While we try to batten down a few stupidities, they turn into rabbits and we finish trying to batten down dozens. Let them all come; invite them all. Unwanted thoughts dislike being invited to the party so much, they rarely come.

* For a full list of Dr Weekes' cassettes and recordings, and information on where to obtain them, see p. 425.

OCCUPATION AND DEPRESSION

I was talking to a group of nervously ill people in England, and noticed a woman sitting quietly in one corner. She seldom spoke. Her husband had died six months previously and she had but one daughter who lived in London. She was quiet because she was so depressed. Each day was a burden. The housework was done by early morning and then the long empty hours lay ahead.

When the group began discussing how they would help her to be occupied, her face lit up and she came to life. The promise of work did more for that woman than all the anti-depressant drugs and tranquillizers she had taken.

When suitable occupation in the company of other people is found for lonely or depressed people, such medication can often be washed down the sink.

NOT AGAIN!

'It's difficult in setback to remember how well I felt when I was making good progress. How can I shorten the time in a setback? I get feelings like, "I can't go through all that first-line battle stuff again! I really can't!" But I do go through it.'

It's difficult in setback to remember how well one recently felt, because setback itself brings such disappointment. Also, nervous feelings seem to be so much more acute when they have been absent for some time. So much of their sting may have been forgotten that when it returns it can shock!

Shock, fear, exasperation and despair are so normal in setback they are even part of recovery! I like my patients to have setbacks and the experience of learning how to come out of them. The experience gained in coming through each setback absorbs some of the shock of future setbacks and brings heart-warming encouragement. So welcome setback, don't shrink from it.

ROOTED TO THE GROUND

'When I have to stand still even for a short time, I feel as if my feet are rooted to the ground and my body is swaying about.'

Severe tension can bring a feeling of being 'rooted to the ground'. Trying to force a way forward does not help – it acts like a clamp. The answer is to float, not fight. Simply thinking of floating can relax and loosen, and a loosened body can move.

One of my patients – a violinist, who'd not worked for two years – on recovering, was very anxious to get back to playing on the stage. He accepted an engagement and after finishing his solo, bowed, and turned to leave. He couldn't budge. His right foot was clamped to the floor. He began to panic and thought, 'What would Dr Weekes say now! She'd say float, so I've got to float!' But he couldn't move his foot. It was clamped to the floor by a ball of chewing gum. Floating can dissolve tension, but not gum.

FEAR OF OPEN HEIGHTS

Many people are afraid of them. To look down many storeys over an open balcony needs nerve and a strong stomach. I always get a clutching hand in mine. Treating such dislike is comparable to treating dislike of being in a lift. I never worry my patients about trying to overcome fear of lifts unless they need to use them often and the alternative is climbing long flights of stairs.

However, fear of open heights can be embarrassing; for example, when visiting a friend in his penthouse. So here's a suggestion (I do this myself): as you look over the balcony (or cliff-edge or whatever) take the usual deep breaths and let them out very slowly and really *look* down with open eyes, head forward – no head-back, narrow-eyed look! Doing this, I can even look out the window of a plane as it banks to land.

AN ADEQUATE MEDICAL EXAMINATION

I have sometimes been asked by a nervously ill person what I consider to be an adequate examination. When I was a general practitioner, an adequate examination meant asking a patient to remove most of his clothes and then examining him on the couch: his hair, eyes, tongue, mouth, palpating the neck, looking at the hands, feeling the pulse, listening to the heart and chest, palpating the breasts and abdomen, testing arteries in legs and feet, examining reflexes, taking blood pressure and examining urine. Any further tests made would depend on the results of such an examination. That would be an adequate examination and would not take so long if practised often enough to become routine.

BLOOD PRESSURE TABLETS

I am writing this short warning because the dose prescribed (especially of a beta-blocker) for so many people with high blood pressure is too heavy. On a too heavy dose, they can feel apathetic, lethargic – even depressed; have 'weak turns', dragging, heavy legs and a tendency to stagger. They can also have pains and a feeling of weakness across the chest – mimicking angina. Too often the victim mistakes these symptoms for 'a bad 'heart' and suffers unnecessarily while he drags himself from day to day.

Because beta-blockers slow the heart rate, they are sometimes prescribed for the anxiety state. Obviously the dose should be carefully monitored, otherwise it could complicate rather than help.

UPSETTING IRRITATION: THUMPING ON THE BED!

A man wrote, 'A friend visited me while I was ill. As he talked he thumped the end of my bed with his fist – a heavy thump. Should I have put up with this (accepted it), or should I have told him to please stop. Would that have been running away, not accepting?'

It would have been wise, not running away. There's no need to be martyred unnecessarily. When sensitized (as this man was) nervous reaction to an irritant can be extreme. If a thumping fist (dripping tap, ticking clock, talkative neighbour) can't be stopped, try relaxing toward it and actually listening to it. This works.

AFTER THE BIRTH OF MY BABY!

So many mothers say, 'It all began after the birth of my baby!' Sometimes the exertion of childbirth, with the possible upset in glandular balance, and the work and loss of sleep a new baby entails, are enough to lead to depletion and depression.

Any mother, when depleted, can become afraid of harming her children – especially a young baby, so trusting, so dependent.

The thought can naturally flash in the tired mind, 'Wouldn't it be awful if I hurt my baby!' And even to 'Perhaps I really wound!'

Unfortunately, some of these mothers are told by their therapists that they are aggressive types. They are *not* aggressive types; they are simply passing through an obsessive phase which anyone could have in similar circumstances. Once more, cure lies in glimpsing the obsession as ONLY A THOUGHT IN A TIRED MIND MAKING AN EXAGGERATED IMPRESSION ON A SENSITIZED BODY.

DREADING HOT WEATHER

Dilation of blood vessels in hot weather (to allow for cooling) can bring symptoms similar to those of nervous illness: flushed face, throbbing head, sweating, perhaps thumping heart and even fatigue. These symptoms may dupe a nervously fatigued, or nervously ill person, into thinking that his nerves are once more 'in a bad way'. Even if he finally understands the cause – hot weather – he may come to so dread the heat, he encourages the symptoms.

Some nervously ill people complain that cold weather also increases awareness of nervous symptoms. The effects of weather, hot or cold, should be understood and since we can't change the weather, we know what to do!

A HUSBAND'S HELP

A woman who had been agoraphobic for 12 years asked if she would ever function on her own without her husband's help. Answer: she won't until she tries. Twelve years is a long time to be without confidence. To change that situation she must change herself – and soon. She must not wait for confidence to come to her; it won't.

She must face taking those first tottering steps holding her own hand, not her husband's! And she must try to be not too discouraged by failure. Of course, she will fail sometimes, so why waste time being impressed by it!

She must practise, practise, practise, the way I have consistently taught her in my books (for her, especially *Simple, Effective Treatment of Agoraphobia*) and cassettes (again, for her, the cassette, *Moving to Freedom*, in which I go through panic with her). It's all there. At least when she decides to practise without her husband, she will be pointing herself in the right direction at last: toward recovery.

LIVING WITH A NERVOUSLY ILL RELATIVE

People who live with a nervously ill relative need short spells away from the tension. It's useless to simply keep making and breaking resolutions about being patient. The binding tension that can follow no more than a plaintive request from the sick relative can shatter all such resolutions. Spells away, however short, are the remedy, but more easily prescribed than obtained.

FEAR OF ILLNESS

Most people become neither seriously ill nor die young. So the odds are in our favour. However, no nervously ill person should live in anxious doubt about his health. He should immediately consult his doctor about any suspicious symptom and so get peace of mind and he must not think that by doing this he is being hypochondriacal. He is being sensible.

Also, the death we fear when young may hold no fears as we grow older. When old, simply doing the ordinary jobs that mean living can become an effort and so death gradually loses its terrors; indeed to many it may seem like a release. Even the manner of dying need not be feared. I have seen so many die peacefully, unaware that they were dying. When my mother was ill, my brothers and their children came to see her and afterwards she laughingly said, 'The old sillies! My birthday was last Saturday, not today!' She didn't realize she was ill, and yet she died that same week. She had said to me some years earlier, 'I am not afraid of dying. I am just a little afraid of how I will die.' She died in her sleep. So, don't waste the young years worrying about the old years to come.

HOW WILL I KNOW WHEN I'M CURED?

When you can live in peace with the memory of what you have been through and if, when times of stress bring back your old symptoms, you can accept these and not let them upset you too much, not let them disrupt your life, then you can say you are cured.

Of course, being cured does not mean having a constantly peaceful body. Life must always hold some stress to which one's body may respond with some upsetting symptoms, so don't search for the impossible – calm, perfect calm, always!

Recovery means that although symptoms can return under stress, there is a deep inner feeling of peace because the symptoms have come to no longer matter. Nothing can completely take away this feeling and it comes only when past successful experiences have become your insulation against despair. In other words, you may have to come through setbacks successfully many times before you can finally face one calmly, knowing so well how to cope with it because *it no longer matters!*

CONSTANT NAUSEA

Treating constant nausea is difficult, because so often it is the result of constant anxiety. When the mind is at peace nausea can go surprisingly quickly. A chronically nauseated, nervously ill woman under great stress was persuaded to take a holiday. She said that from feeling too nauseated to even look at food, she ate hungrily on the aeroplane. From then on during the holiday she ate well, with no nausea. However on the return plane journey the nausea returned. This showed her clearly how closely it was related to stress.

Of course everyone can't have a holiday to relieve nausea; however there are a few other remedies to try. First, check constipation; this occurs frequently in nervous illness, when the sufferer is too agitated to take enough time on the toilet and perhaps does not drink enough fluid or eat much food.

In nervous illness the tongue may be coated and sour (often aggravated by tranquillizers). The tongue should be cleaned with a soft toothbrush and then the mouth cleansed with a mild mouthwash: glycothymol works well and is pleasant.

If the doctor has prescribed a tranquillizer for nausea, it should be taken half an hour before the main meal.

Also, a nervously ill person should not try to face a big meal sitting with the family. He usually has more success managing a small meal in private (if this can be arranged). Eating with others at the table, especially if the conversation is noisy, demands a great deal of effort from a very tired person. Also, it may be less effort to pick at food during the day, instead of facing a set meal: a dish of nuts, fruit, dried fruit, cubes of cheese, biscuits and so on, in different rooms. Of course, there is the old stand-by – egg and milk beaten together with added flavouring.

If the nervously ill person is eating poorly, vitamin supplements are essential, but not in massive does. Too many can be as dangerous as too few; for example, too much Vitamin B_1 can overstimulate.

Tablets are prescribed for nausea; for example, thiethylterazime (called Torecan in Australia). Unfortunately anti-nausea tablets can sometimes cause drowsiness. The good news is that when stress goes, nausea goes with it. I do not worry my patients about low-cholesterol diets while they're trying to recover an appetite. Even when well, moderation in all things!

UNNECESSARY WORRY

Carrying worry around is a hangover from the time when there was too much genuine worry, perhaps a too rapid succession of worries.

Worry can vary from being a tension-headache to being simply a dull, rather muzzy feeling in the head, rather like a threatening headache. One woman said that although she knew there was nothing now to worry about, she still played the 'worry-record' and felt sure that if she searched diligently enough she'd find some worry somewhere.

The worry habit is encouraged by staying indoors too much. Sometimes to simply walk through the front door into the light, into activity, is enough to alert the worrier to the greyness of the worry-cloud enveloping him. He can then appreciate that his worry is a physical state rather than a reality.

While such small shocks help, bigger shocks (like going on holiday) help even more. Tension is eased and a habit broken.

For 'chronic worriers' who cannot have a holiday I recommend working out-of-doors; the feeling of space above can lift the pressing ceiling of worry-tension.

TENSION AND OBSESSION

'When I am with my doctor, I can relax and believe all is right – that I will never harm anyone wilfully – but when I leave him the obsession returns.'

When the doctor relieved her tension, and she relaxed, she could think more flexibly – think 'around corners' – and see her obsession as simply an idea that she could dismiss.

Although temporarily eased by the doctor, the tension underlying obsession is great indeed and could grip with its old force as soon as this woman thought again – as she invariably must – of the obsession. Indeed, tension could grip before she left the doctor's office. She would probably then think, 'Oh God! Here it is again! And after all the doctor said! There's no hope for me!'

The return of an obsession, after thinking it lost, can bring shock that feels like a physical blow. A doctor should explain this. Understanding obsession and how it works and then practising 'glimpsing' can save months of suffering and finally cure. I described 'glimpsing' in Chapter Three.

HOW TO KNOW WHEN YOU ARE NORMAL?

'I have been nervously ill since childhood, so how will I know when I'm better? I don't know what being normal means;

most people aim to be as they were, but I have no guidelines.'

This woman should work on without analysing her feelings too closely, without considering whether they are normal or not; without wondering, 'Now what did they mean by that?', or 'What did I mean by that? Was that a normal reaction?' She must try not to be critical of her reactions; she should give them the signal, 'Full steam ahead!'

Being normal simply means her being less self-critical, less self-aware and more at ease with people.

As she goes forward without too much introspection, normality will embrace her gently. She will be at ease.

She can take heart. Few nervously ill people remain as they were before their illness. Character strengthens as difficulties are overcome. Recovery is a new experience for all.

So this woman need not worry about recognizing normality in herself. She should not try to search for it, but live from day to day letting normality come to her. She will recognize it because she will gradually feel less tense, more at ease.

GOING FOR A JOB

Should a person who has recovered from nervous illness mention the past when being interviewed for a job? A woman recently telephoned from the United States saying that although she was a good floral arranger (she had owned her own shop), she could not get a job in her home town because rumours about her having been nervously ill had spread quickly in the florist world. She said that for the first few days in a new job all would be well, then the freeze would start. Unfortunately, few people can understand nervous illness until they have experienced it.

Having been nervously ill is a very private affair; so keep it private when you apply for a job. You need not feel guilty. Experience gained in recovering the hard way – and mine is the hard way – builds character. Anyone can be tricked into becoming nervously ill; often it's just chance that some are and some aren't.

If we talked more freely about nervous illness, how much less mysterious it would be! There is no bogyman manipulating people into 'it', only certain natural laws working automatically and which can be reversed when we know how to reverse them. So don't feel guilty when you keep your business to yourself; perhaps feel just a little wiser, more mature, than those around.

WISHING IT WOULD ALL GO AWAY

'I wish it would all go away. I'm tired of battling with these thoughts!'

There is no 'it'; there is only his habit of thinking, grooved by mental fatigue. What he tries to forget one minute, habit and fatigue will present again the next. Although he can switch attention if something important demands it, when the demand passes he quickly remembers the 'battling' and is caught once more in the old habit.

I repeat again and again, that recovery lies in accepting strange thoughts as part of ordinary thinking – especially repeated thought. Constant repetition can itself be upsetting, although the thought may not be strange.

This man should not think, 'I mustn't think that!' and then shy away from the thoughts, hoping they will go. He must understand that in his present state of self-awareness he hasn't a hope of forgetting them. He should relax toward them, think them willingly. When he does this, tension will ease, the 'grooves' melt and the habit gradually lift. This is the only way.

STOPPING 'HORRIBLE' THOUGHTS ABOUT LOVED ONES

'My psychologist said I must stop these horrible thoughts coming. Is that the way to deal with my problem?'

No. While this man fears these thoughts so much, how can he stop them? He should, as I advise so often, understand that THEY ARE ONLY THOUGHTS, HOWEVER HORRIBLE and let them come.

The writer of the letter added that the thoughts were about those he loved and that it hurt so much to know that he could think this way.

So many nervously ill people have the most bizarre thoughts particularly about those they love, because this hurts most, and in a state of sensitization and fatigue, a sufferer may deliberately probe to see how horrible his thoughts can be. This is so common in nervous illness, it seems part of an expected pattern. Its only significance is that the sufferer, being so suggestible, can't resist testing his own suggestibility. How cruelly can he think? How crazy can he be? How much more is there to be frightened of?

As I say so often, a person suffering this way should practise seeing his thoughts for what they are: thoughts established, not because of their truth, but because of the intense, fearful reaction they bring to a sensitized body. And he should understand that they may return from time to time even after he has lost fear of them. Habits take time to break. But when thoughts no longer matter, what harm if they do sometimes return.

Essential Help for your Nerves

With acceptance the time comes when the sufferer suddenly thinks gleefully, 'The darn things don't matter any more! They just don't matter! It doesn't matter whether I think them or not!' We lose upsetting thoughts *by drawing their teeth, not by trying to stop their biting*.

GROUP THERAPY

I've been communicating with groups of nervously ill people in Australia, Great Britain, America, Africa and Canada. Many members seem satisfied with their group and are making progress. Yesterday, the organizer of a group telephoned and said that her members inspired each other to get moving and that the progress of some was incredible.

Providing a group has positive-minded members, it can give great support and motivation, especially to lonely people. A group of pessimists who 'can't do this', 'can't do that', is of little help. The majority of group members I have met are optimists; however, if you join a group, don't feel obliged to stay with it if you find it unsatisfactory.

Anyone considering starting a group should be on guard against feeling power. It's so easy to feel power when at the head of a group of nervous, vulnerable, suggestible, nervously ill people. The leader of a group should always stay humbled by his own experiences and always see him, or her, self, as a friend and helper, never as a particularly gifted therapist and certainly never as God. One therapist said to me, 'How do you stop yourself from feeling like God?' I think that illustrates my meaning. Beware of that trap.

CAN WE FORGIVE OURSELVES?

The nearest we can come to forgiving ourselves is to realize that we are different now from that person who transgressed and that we would not make the same mistake today. Life demands mistakes and demands that we remember them.

So we must be philosophical about our past mistakes. And that is about as close as any of us can get to forgiving ourselves.

RECOVERED FROM NERVOUS ILLNESS, BUT NOT ENJOYING LIVING ALONE OR GOING OUT

Living alone is difficult for some (it's not easy to laugh on one's own!) and for a person who has been nervously ill it can be especially difficult because she (a woman made this complaint) may still carry 'the shadow of the shadow' – a mixture of memory and some hangover-depletion.

Also, she may feel cheated of time by her illness and may, when out, be too aware of needing to enjoy herself, of having to make up for all those lost months. So, she may try too hard, perhaps expect too much.

Nature will restore vitality in her own time, if this woman cooperates by not trying for enjoyment too earnestly and is prepared to let more time pass and not watch her progress too closely while she waits.

WHY DO THINGS LOOK DIFFERENT?

'Why is it that when I visit a familiar place – but perhaps not seen for some time – it looks and seems different, although it hasn't really changed? I keep saying to whoever's with me, "Does it look different to you? Are you sure it doesn't look different?".'

A nervously ill person lives so much in his own thoughts, that when he visits a place he has not seen for some time, this change in his surroundings can almost forcibly draw him out of himself, make him notice the outside world. This experience is the strangeness he feels, not so much the place. For a moment everything may look clean, almost 'just washed' – certainly different – because he's probably looking at it intently for the first time in months.

This is all part of recovery. Isn't that good?

IS THERE A COMPLETE CURE?

It would surely be difficult for a nervously ill person to suffer as he has and not sometimes recoil at the memory. For as long as memory brings suffering, doubting complete recovery is natural.

Recovery means being able to look full-faced at memory, prepared to accept any suffering it may bring. Complete cure does not necessarily mean absence of symptoms, although it can. It means knowing how to cope with the symptoms stress may present, at any time, any place.

Being able to cope is not only possible, it is inevitable, when recovery has been earned by the sufferer's own effort based on understanding.

HYPOGLYCAEMIA

During the last decade some therapists have stressed the importance of hypoglycaemia in causing nervous illness. I have seen it do this occasionally. An unsuspecting and normally healthy person, after eating little breakfast, could have a spell of weakness, trembling, perhaps sweating before lunch and mistakenly think he is about to die, or at least have a heart attack. Unless the innocence of the attack were explained to him, he could perhaps become afraid of going out alone 'for fear of having a spell' and so perhaps develop agoraphobia.

Hypoglycaemia means low bloodsugar – too little glucose in the blood. Glucose is our source of energy, so naturally with a too low supply we can feel all the symptoms mentioned above.

But, while blood may not have enough glucose, the liver has it stored as glycogen which it breaks down into glucose to meet the blood's demand; so that rest alone (while the liver does its work) will remedy low blood sugar.

However, the sufferer wants quick relief (before he 'dies'!) and this comes with eating. The instinct is to reach for something sweet; however, protein (for example, a piece of cheese, banana) should be the main choice supplemented with a *little* sugar. Too much sweet stimulates the pancreas to secrete more insulin and so the attack may recur later.

Hypoglycaemia is not serious in a normally healthy person and many, many people have had at least one attack. Some causes are: (1) not enough protein for breakfast – the dashed-off cup of coffee, slammed front door, the 'shakes' before lunch (the 'I never eat breakfast!' syndrome); (2) stress stimulating the pancreas to excessive secretion of insulin – anyone under stress, especially the nervously ill, can have attacks of hypoglycaemia even soon after a meal. This can puzzle the sufferer. He need wonder no longer, (3) a diet too rich in sugar – this also overstim-ulates the pancreas to secrete insulin; (4) being prediabetic or diabetic; (5) post-operative – an operation on the stomach in par-ticular; (6) diseases of the pancreas.

A nervously ill person reading this could immediately think, 'Perhaps I have a disease of my pancreas or am diabetic!' To ease these fears he should have his urine tested for glucose. The five-hour glucose tolerance test is very popular today; however, recognizing that stress can stimulate secretion of insulin and cause hypoglycaemia, a simple urine test for glucose is, in my opinion, adequate for a nervously ill person who fears diabetes. Clinitix for testing is sold by the pharmacist.

RELAXING MENTALLY

'You say so often "loosen and accept" and I can loosen physically by taking deep breaths and letting them out slowly and then by relaxing my muscles, particularly chest and abdominal muscles. This I do conscientiously and deliberately. But how do I loosen mentally? I know that physical relaxation helps to relax mentally, but what can I do *mentally* to bring loosening? What thoughts should I think to be able to relax mentally?'

Feeling constant 'mental tension', despite attempts at physi-cal relaxation, sends so many reaching for a tranquillizer, cigarette, alcohol. Tension from stress can be so severe that the slightest touch of extra tension (perhaps a mere flicker of anxiety) can put muscles into a binding clinch: the iron-band around the scalp. The iron-band is sometimes mistaken for mental tension because it seems to tighten further with each stressful thought.

When this man asks what to think to help him loosen men-tally, he really means what to think to lessen muscular tension that feels like mental tension. There is no such thing as mental tension.

Some people have described how, when in a moment of what they called 'great mental tension', their thoughts have seemed to recede to the back of their head – back, back, back! They thought that if they did not hold on grimly and resist that backward drift, they would go 'over the edge' and never come back. They were never sure where they would recede to because their imagination baulked at looking clearly over that edge, where they suspected insanity might lie. Few realized they were feeling no more than a severe spasm of muscular tension. Brains may seem dull, muzzy, but they do not tense.

This man is really asking what he should think about in order to comfort himself and so help his muscles relax. If he is upset only by 'the state he is in' – that is, of his continuous waking early and feeling fearful for no special reason (as I suspect) – I suggest that he switch on the light and read this book. There should be comfort there.

WILL I FAINT?

The fear of fainting haunts many nervously ill people. When questioned, they admit that although they have 'felt like it', they have never actually fainted.

What is so terrible about fainting? I've done it many times. It seems to be my reaction to intense physical pain. However, I can always manage to find a safe place to fall before I go right off; ringing in the ears gives a good warning.

For some nervously ill, there is the added fear of 'making a scene' in front of other people. What matter if people see one faint? All the better: there'll be someone there to help, if help is needed. Actually, little help is needed, because in the horizontal (fainting) position, circulation rights itself and the victim revives.

On questioning nervously ill people who say that they have fainted, I usually find some contributing cause; for example, they may have been standing still for a long time. A fall in blood supply to the brain can cause fainting.

If only the nervously ill person who fears fainting could faint and get it over! Familiarity breeds contempt, even of fainting. It's the great unknown that frightens. And, as I mentioned earlier, before fainting one usually has enough warning to position oneself safely. Once, when I was about to faint, a friend with me said 'Quickly, tell me what I have to do! I haven't a clue!' I had time to tell her to do nothing.

A BINDING AWARENESS OF SELF: INWARD THINKING

A person may have recovered from much of his nervous illness to find that he has developed a consciousness of himself – of his thoughts, actions – which bewilders, alarms and exhausts. He delays his own recovery by a too fierce, too tense recoil from this self-awareness; he feels imprisoned within himself and makes the mistake of struggling to be free, trying to force self-forgetfulness.

Little can be forced successfully in nervous illness, least of all forgetfulness of self. The only way to lose this inward-thinking (as I call it) is *not* to recoil from it, *to let it come and accept it as part of ordinary thinking;* to accept it as part of ordinary, normal awareness, however stifling it may seem, however 'crazy', devastating, exhausting, frightening. ACCEPT IT ALL. WORK WITH IT THERE, WILLINGLY!

I know that some fear that if they do this they will become more firmly entrenched in the habit. THEY WON'T. I ASSURE THEM.

If they let inward-thinking (and this includes self-awareness) come with utter acceptance, the habit will gradually lose its significance and *they will be free*. I do not mean that they will never think inwardly – we all do unconsciously some of the time – but they will not see it as unusual or frustrating. Its presence will not matter any more.

If a former sufferer has been free of inward-thinking (especially for a long time), and then, one day, feels menaced by its return, he should try not to recoil in shock. Once more he should relax, go toward it, let it come, remembering that if he does this with utter acceptance, the habit will once more 'mizzle' as it did in the past.

A student described his sudden insight into inward-thinking. One evening, a neighbour stood talking to him while standing in the doorway swinging a lantern. As the student watched the man's mouth move and the lantern swing, his thoughts as usual, kept reverting to himself. He was so distraught by this that he hardly heard what the man was saying. Then suddenly his thoughts seemed to revert more lightly, with less tension. He thought, 'It doesn't really matter what I think when I do this! I could just as well keep thinking "Tick!" This is only a habit of thinking back to myself. Only a habit!' He said it was almost as if a light suddenly shone in the room, and his spirits leapt as he realized that any outside interest would be enough to free him from the habit.

The next day when the habit returned he said it seemed as if a grey curtain would descend for a while and then lift again. He recognized the curtain as fatigue and was elated, because during the moment of its lifting he could glimpse so well that he would recover. A few days later some friends in another state invited him to visit them and he knew that if he accepted the change, the curtain would lift very quickly and would stay lifted.

He chose to remain where he was, working on his own with his thoughts on himself. He wanted to prove to himself that he could recover without distraction. He wanted to know that if the habit returned in the future, he would not have to depend on change or diversion, to lose it again. He stayed and proved his point. He had released the tension that bound his thoughts to himself. He had 'rolled with the punches' and recovered.

Some therapists' ignorance of inward-thinking is tragic because, as I have explained, it can be cured. A lecturer at an Australian university treated, for two years, a woman with inward-thinking. He used psychoanalysis. Finally he told her he could neither understand her condition nor cure her. However, he said that an American psychiatrist would be visiting the university and that he might be able to help her. After treating her for six months, this visiting doctor said, 'I don't understand your illness either!' This ignorance was tragic because it meant years of unnecessary suffering for her. She was finally cured by the understanding and acceptance I taught her.

FLATULENCE MAY NOT BE NERVOUS

'I have suffered from flatulence since childhood but it has worsened during the last years. I am now 70. I have most of the other symptoms of nervous depletion. I faithfully carry out your directions of facing, accepting, floating and letting time pass, but I still suffer from flatulence.

'The doctors at the hospital say there is no physical reason and that I am a wind-swallower. They offer no cure. One suggested that I hold a cork between my teeth after each meal. This, they said, would prevent me swallowing air. I've tried this for a long time and it doesn't work. I have wind continually whatever I eat and however much I chew my food. So I have begun to think it must be nervous.'

So many doctors talk about wind-swallowing. People don't swallow wind for the fun of it; they do it mainly because their stomach feels uncomfortable. In my opinion, the discomfort comes first and brings the urge to swallow. Certainly swallowing air increases discomfort which again encourages more swallowing. Holding a cork between the teeth after meals is a favourite and futile prescription, which leads only to a lot of dribbling and more discomfort. What is one supposed to do with the dribble if not swallow it? And with it, more air!

The causes of flatulence are so many, it's daunting to begin to discuss them. In middle-aged and older people, perhaps one of the commonest causes is oesophageal reflux. As we age, the normally tight sphincter between our swallowing tube (oesophagus) and our stomach may become lax, especially if we are overweight, so that when we stoop – for example, to tie shoes, clean the bath – the acid contents of our stomach may rise into our oesophagus and cause heartburn. If the area (at the base of the breastbone) is frequently bathed with acid it may become inflamed and hurt as food passes through it, especially 'acid' or spicy food: curry, pineapple, fruit cake, tomatoes, alcohol, fizzy drinks and so on.

Flatulence can be nervous; our stomach is our most sympathetic organ; it weeps when other organs are in trouble. So, to treat nervous flatulence, any outstanding problem should be resolved if possible. This can be difficult in one's seventies. That peaceful old age we are promised when young is a mirage for many. Old age can bring so many problems – and when we feel too tired to cope!

So, while flatulence can certainly be nervous, there are many other organic causes which should be checked.

CHAPTER 6

✻

Talks with Patients

FIRST PATIENT

Watching For the Build-Up

A nervously ill person is greatly influenced by his mood of the moment because his body reacts so quickly and so acutely to it. The man in the following interview said he'd had a wonderful day, got up next morning and still felt wonderful but that when he turned to open a window – flash! Unreality smote! He couldn't work this out. He'd gone to bed feeling peaceful, had wakened peaceful, so why the sudden flash?

He did not realize that under the feeling of peace, his body was still sensitized and nervously fatigued. Physically damaged nerves can take up to six months to heal, so why shouldn't sensitized nerves take time also. They do. His nerves were still ready to respond too quickly and too intensely to the slightest shock – even a sudden turn that may have brought a feeling of 'floatiness' in the head.

At the time of this experience, this man was on holiday. His nerves had felt peaceful during the day he mentioned because nothing had occurred to aggravate them, test them; but as soon as he got a slight shock (he may have turned to the window very quickly) sensitization reared its head and showed itself in a flash. Nervous illness takes a lot of understanding, doesn't it? Recovery is a question of enough time passing for habit and reaction to lose their grip.

The same man said he could be under enormous tension at the office with his head feeling as if pressed in a vice and yet, if something caught his attention, even though it brought tense concentration, the vice-like grip would ease and the tension disappear. But, although he was no longer so afraid of the symptoms of nervous illness, he still watched for the 'build-up', especially the brain-fag.

THE PATIENT (THE SAME MAN): 'Doctor, although I'm getting better I have a funny lost feeling. How can this be, when I know I'm recovering?'

DOCTOR: 'You feel lost because you are no longer constantly occupied with watching your symptoms and worrying about them. It's a long time since you had no symptoms to worry about; of course you will feel strange for a while.'

PATIENT: 'It's interesting, that although I'm no longer as afraid of the symptoms, I still watch for that build-up, especially the brain-fag part.'

DOCTOR: 'The brain-fag comes very quickly at the moment.'

PATIENT: 'Within seconds.'

DOCTOR: 'Looking for a build-up is part of recovery. This is why so many feel bewildered by recovery.'

PATIENT: 'I can understand people fighting against it, because when the feeling comes I feel as if I will be lost for ever unless I do fight it.'

DOCTOR: 'Don't try to keep a "hold" on yourself. You don't come back to being yourself that way. Let go and float up. I say *up* to, not *back* to, because always remember you go forward, forward in thought, never backward. Never try to scramble back to where you think you were before you were ill, or even before you had a particular setback. Always float forward; always onward. Trying to get back is like Lot's wife. Beware that pillar of salt.

'Also, instant recovery from nervous illness is very rare (although I have seen it). Usually you have to pack in much more normal living before you can feel normal and know that the feeling is established, not just grasped momentarily. You need so much ordinary living to be able to relax in it with assurance. Time must pass; always give it time.

'Also, in the beginning when you first have moments of feeling normal, this feeling can be mixed with other emotions, even elation, and this can be a trap. While you feel elated you can suddenly switch to feeling abnormal again because, naturally, you feel strange feeling elated! It may be a long time since you felt normal, so the feeling may seem strange, even abnormal.'

PATIENT: 'You're right, doctor. When I'm happy, for instance, at the club, I suddenly think, "I shouldn't feel like this!" And I almost feel guilty because I'm feeling well. So my heart sinks again and there seems no way out.

'And yet, I'm feeling so much better. I'm not over-reacting the way I was. I'm floating up gently. The funny thing is, I'm even a bit afraid to be happy about that!'

DOCTOR (LAUGHING): 'You become too excited and your mind switches back immediately to your illness when you were agitated and you feel drawn back into the quagmire. Don't be oppressed by this, don't be oppressed by the strangeness of any feeling, particularly of feeling happy. It must feel strange.

Pass through, on. Recognize feeling guilty because you are happy as one of those flash-moments through which you must always pass.'

PATIENT: 'I think this feeling of being lost is mostly when I'm tired and can't talk to myself convincingly.'

DOCTOR: 'You are right. Your body has responded to anxiety too intensely for so long, you have to be only mildly anxious now to feel a strong undercurrent of apprehension.

'You may ask yourself what on earth you are anxious about and will you ever stop apprehending. It's difficult to believe you will, but living with utter acceptance of all the strangeness will eventually bring enough relaxation and freedom from stress to finally bring peace. So, on your way!'

A Later Session with the Same Patient

PATIENT: 'It's so difficult to stay peaceful, even when I know what to do!'

DOCTOR: 'To recover, you have to accept that the human body is like a machine. It is fantastic and works marvellously for us; however, it can be strained by too heavy a load. Although you said that in your youth you felt like a god, eager to achieve, your body knew you were achieving the wrong way – too much impetuous ardour, not enough balance, not enough time for contemplation or rest. Too much, "On Stanley, on!" If you are prepared to accept that even *you* have a limit, you will be ready to listen and learn. Also there is a way to placate your hurt ego. You can think, "I'm going to become a better fellow out of this!" What's more, you will be.'

PATIENT: 'Does depression come out of being so concerned with oneself?'

DOCTOR: 'Depression is a form of exhaustion. When anxious

self-concern is frequent it is certainly exhausting and so can bring depression. If you were consistently concerned about someone else, you could also become emotionally drained and consequently depressed. Normally we keep our stores of vitality replenished by day to day uplifting experiences; but when nervously depleted, our feelings are not as easily uplifted, so we miss this daily recharging. It's like a car: if the battery is used to much, the headlights and self-starter fail. Our battery can be depleted in so many ways. We can leave the switch on while we toss and turn at night worrying because we are not getting enough sleep to be ready for tomorrow.'

PATIENT: 'How do you explain the peace of mind I had last night? I went to bed at 2.30 a.m. I lay peacefully in bed and was asleep in five minutes. I woke at 8 this morning feeling great. Did I wake like this because I'd just had five hours peaceful sleep?'

DOCTOR: 'Only partly, but mostly because you are understanding more and recovering. However, recovery will still take time and tomorrow morning may not be as peaceful. You must accept this with good grace. If you had to go into a crisis at work tomorrow, your head would probably feel dull again and the old iron band would grip and you'd think "That three weeks holiday hasn't done any good at all!" ' (He'd just had three weeks holiday.) 'Don't despair if this happens. Simply accept that more time must pass. That's all. The holiday has done its work. You can't estimate the amount of good it's done. The good is there. When you go back to the familiar scenes of suffering, the suffering will not seem quite as close as it was before you went away. Even that short respite from suffering will allow you to look *down* upon it, to understand and accept it with a little less agitation and despair.

'Understanding and willing acceptance are still the same old magic you must use now. Don't expect too much and so add disappointment to the picture. Just give it time.

'You will still have to think as slowly as your tired mind allows. Try not to become impatient, angry, with yourself. Think, "All right! All right! I'll go through with this. I'll take it slowly and quietly. I'm not going to thrash my battery." Tread water without adding disappointment and despair.'

PATIENT: 'If I'm given some bad news when I go back, how will I cope with that?'

DOCTOR: 'Let the first shock pass. Don't act on the moment's reaction. Let the reaction spend itself. Let your body do what it wants to and don't fight to try to save yourself from it. Let the reaction come. Accept it. You will find, that after you go through the initial shock, as your body calms down, you will think of ways to cope.'

PATIENT: 'I know I blow things up out of proportion; my wife says, "How can you be so stupid!" I say, "I don't know. I wish I did!" For a long time I couldn't bring myself to accept that I, so confident, had lost myself. Now I can accept it.'

DOCTOR: 'And also being a man of action, you want to do something about it quick smart! It is difficult for you to accept that you get better quicker by doing nothing active about it. Actually, although you appear to do nothing, you are doing something very positive and very difficult: you are accepting the state you are in. This is tremendous. It has taken you months, hasn't it, to understand? You wanted a switch to turn off the suffering quickly. You all search for an outside switch – a new tablet, a new doctor.'

PATIENT: 'It's the hardest part for me to master, but it's beginning to come. I don't know what to do about the Serepax. Should I start cutting down now?'

DOCTOR: 'Not yet. I don't want you complicating recovery by having withdrawal symptoms at this stage. And when you decide to stop taking them, don't do it suddenly. Anyhow, I'll help you with that.' (I had not prescribed the Serepax.)

'You will know you are getting better as you begin to handle stress without so much reaction. Certainly some stress will come at work but you will find you can sail through it. In other words your nerves will have regained some of their normal insulation – they will not be so easily aroused.'

Final Interview with the Same Patient

PATIENT: 'I'm still afraid to think, "Look, you're on top of the world!" even though I feel like it.'

DOCTOR: 'You can think of it, providing you're prepared to be afraid of thinking it! What does it matter if you are afraid to think it? That kind of fear is all part of getting better. Up one minute and down the next! Up and down! What the heck! Why worry about the downs? They pass. When you can accept tomorrow as it comes, you are recovering all the time. Acceptance that tomorrow may not be so good alone relieves some tension. Acceptance means that you are no longer thinking, "This is wonderful, but I wonder what I'll be like tomorrow!"'

PATIENT: 'What came over me on my holiday? Why did I slip back, Doctor? Why did I slip right back when I was doing so well? After that second week when I started to go to pieces, you said on the telephone for me to keep occupied normally: to take drives, have fun, lead the kind of life I would normally lead on such a holiday. I did and I started to pick up and then, after one bad night, I started to worry again because I wanted to be so much better by the end of the three weeks when I knew I had to go home and face work again. So, I panicked. After two weeks when I thought I was getting better, down I went.'

DOCTOR: 'You did it to yourself, you know, by putting a time limit on getting better. You gave yourself that constant tension; can you see that?'

PATIENT: 'Yes and I was so depressed by the setback. By the third week I was really down, worse than when I first arrived.'

DOCTOR: 'You sought to relieve stress and yet in your ignorance you created it with too much anxious watching, expectation. You did not let time pass, you know.'

PATIENT: 'My biggest problem is that the sickness I've had over the last couple of years has been because of a tremendous amount of pressure – strain and worry with the business. I felt it as a persistent pounding the minute I walked into the office. There were only very short times for enjoyment and rest; I was so hassled.'

DOCTOR: 'Need you go back to that pace?'

PATIENT: 'No, I've got it running now. I'd close it all up before I'd go back to that! I'm not going to run away from it, but I'm going to use my brains now; I'm going to delegate more. I know now that other people can do the job as well as I can. I used to lie in bed and think about the problems until 3 in the morning and the only way I could get relief was to take alcohol. I think I've done a pretty good job these last 12 months getting out of that one.'

DOCTOR: 'You've got more out of today than on any previous visit. I think you have the hang of it now.'

PATIENT: 'I think I have, if for only one reason. I've always thought of an interval ahead like, "Another month!" Then with the holidays coming up. I'd think, "By the end of the holiday I'll be okay!" Now I've come down to realize the truth. I went to Honolulu for three weeks and that didn't cure me. I went to Miami for two weeks and that didn't cure. I went to Sydney for two weeks and that didn't cure me either. Now I know I can't say I'll be cured by a special time. I'm going back to the farm for the rest of the holiday and I hope I'll be a bit better but I don't expect to be *that* much better and I'm ready to accept even that.'

DOCTOR: 'You've got the right idea at last. That's what I mean when I say, "Let more time pass." Time is all yours, so be prepared to take it.'

PATIENT: 'But I'm the sort of person, make-up-wise, who can't accept humiliation. This is why I'm successful in business. I don't accept anything as impossible. I couldn't accept that I, of all people, could get into this state. I probably wouldn't be like this if I'd been a different kind of person. I guess I just couldn't accept.'

DOCTOR: 'In the beginning I warned you that you probably wouldn't go back recovered and that you had to accept that. You had to learn that recovery takes its own time and you have to give that to it. It's the old four concepts: face, accept, float and let time pass. Every time you have a setback you should say, "Okay, more time must pass." When you go home, at first you may feel good, at ease, and yet when you get into the office where you expect to still feel better, you may suddenly feel like hell. So what? That particular moment of hell is going to pass. Push the carrot at the end of the stick a little further away and pack that moment, that day, behind you.'

PATIENT: 'But the mornings are still pretty bad.'

DOCTOR: 'So what? They are likely to be bad for some time yet. You've been under tension for a long time. It may still be a gigantic effort to drag your body out of bed in the mornings for a few months yet.'

PATIENT: 'I drink a lot of coffee and smoke a lot. Does that help to cause the tiredness?'

DOCTOR: 'Perhaps a little, but you are young and vital. By this I don't mean that when you are better you should continue drinking a lot of coffee and smoking. I mean that any harm it could do now is as nothing compared with what you do to yourself with your anxiety and fear. Be sure to eat enough nourishing food and leave the rest to time.

'You have to accept that you bashed your nervous system and that it will extract its revenge for a while. You are your nervous system you know, and when it records your emotions in an exaggerated way and quickly, you feel as if your foundation has been shaken. And that's hard to understand, hard to cope with. You're flabbergasted by what you have done to yourself. It's difficult to live for one hour, let alone days, weeks, with a body that can respond so sensitively, even to a passing breeze. You feel, "This is crazy! I must be going mad!" But you aren't. Your nerves are just overdoing their job, too eager to oblige.'

PATIENT: 'When that young girl asked me to play tennis on holiday, I thought, "I'll never be able to handle it!" And the minute I worried about it I felt weak and I went down, down, down and stopped playing. And yet in the afternoon, I went water-skiing and came back and felt so good. But the next morning I was down again. And yet in the afternoon, I played two hours' table tennis. The next day, I couldn't even hold a bat! Oh, God! It's confusing!'

DOCTOR: 'When you felt so good skiing and playing table tennis you thought, "This is it! I've made it!" But you hadn't you know. Instead you should have thought, "Okay, this is good! I'm really enjoying this! What the heck if I feel tired tomorrow. Eventually I'll feel good all the time!"'

PATIENT: 'I really do see at last, doctor. I know where I went wrong.'

This man is fully recovered.

SECOND PATIENT

Trembling Hands

DOCTOR: 'If I had a magic wand, what would you like me to waft away?'

PATIENT: 'The strange feelings I get when I'm handling a cup of tea or a drinking glass. It's when I'm in certain situations; for instance, if I was here on business and you offered me a drink of tea, it would be okay if you offered it in a mug. If it were a flimsy kind of cup, I'd probably use my left hand to pick it up. My right hand would be shaking. That sort of manoeuvre can get carried to an extreme in an emergency.

'If I can rationalize the situation, I can manage. I spend my life watching myself to see that I don't land in too many predicaments. There are dozens of ways you can do a Houdini on yourself and slip out of an embarrassing situation without the obsession being obvious to others.'

DOCTOR: 'The basis of your fear is not of the actual shaking but of making a fool of yourself before other people. If it were the fear of shaking, or fear of the episode that originally caused the shaking (which we've just been discussing) your hand would shake whether you were in company or not.'

PATIENT: 'You're right. It's fear of what people will think.'

DOCTOR: 'There is only one way to cure it permanently. I'll tell you first about a girl who came to me with trembling hands. She'd saved for a long time for a trip to England. She'd been there only a month, when she had a severe shock and her hands began to tremble. She went to many doctors, including neurologists. In her words, she'd been, "All over the place", but nothing stopped the shaking. Her money had run out and as it is not easy to get a job, especially with shaking hands, she returned to Australia.

'I said to her, "You've gone about curing yourself the wrong way by trying to stop your hands from shaking. I want you to let them shake. Don't try to control them. You have to decide what is the most important: letting them shake in front of people and living a normal life or avoiding people because of trembling hands. Your hands don't tremble when you are alone. It's being with people that causes the tension. And that means you are frightened *that they will tremble!*" She said she was prepared to try letting them tremble. I added that she must be prepared for this even if drinking tea with the Queen. She said that that wouldn't be easy because she was afraid she would spill her tea.'

PATIENT: 'So am I! That's just it!'

DOCTOR: 'I know. So I told her to keep the saucer under the cup while she practised. She came back a week later and the shakes had gone. She said, "If only one of those doctors in London had told me that, I could still be there!"

'You see, by tensely trying to control the trembling that was caused by tension, she had simply brought more tension and this is exactly what you are doing. Sometimes you avoid the tension by bluffing yourself – you know, the idea of drinking from a mug and not a cup. But you can't always use a mug.'

PATIENT: 'Are you telling me that I must be prepared to spill the tea?'

DOCTOR: 'Yes. Admit to any onlooker that your hands would probably shake and then be prepared to drink from any kind of container. It's more important for you to lose fear of what others may think than it is for you to go on trying to hide your fear by making excuses, or using a mug instead of a cup.'

PATIENT: 'Must I say straight out that my hands may shake?'

DOCTOR: 'Yes'

PATIENT: 'What if it is a glass with no saucer and worse still, if it's wine!'

DOCTOR: 'Put your handkerchief underneath; use anything.'

PATIENT: 'Even in a restaurant?'

DOCTOR: 'Of course, because that's where you're most frightened.'

PATIENT: 'Don't I know it! When they give you such a little coffee cup at the end of the meal. It's ironic. One place will turn the shakes on and another won't!'

DOCTOR: 'I want you to be prepared to have them turned on, so that eventually it won't matter what the place is like.'

PATIENT: 'I understand. I have a sort of routine of security now. I go to a place where I know the girls will bring the coffee over to me and I won't have to pick it up.'

DOCTOR: 'I want you to be free of all that. And the only way you can do this is to let your hand shake; *let it tremble*. By degrees, if you do this, you will become so used to the trembling, it won't worry you any more. As humans we adapt well and I want you to adapt to having a trembling hand. You haven't adapted so far; you've been running away, trying to cover up. You will find it more difficult to accept when you're tired.'

PATIENT: 'I feel I'm ready to accept while I'm here with you, but being able to do it willingly, as you say, when the time comes and someone's watching me – I don't know. At least I'll try.'

DOCTOR: 'You may not be successful on the first attempt, but if you persevere, I assure you, the shaking will gradually not matter. Especially when you finally feel, deep within yourself, that your *freedom from the fear of it* is more important than *it*.'

THIRD PATIENT

This is a Crazy Business

PATIENT: 'At the level of recovery I reached, with the help of an occasional tranquillizer, I was able to carry on in quite an important position for 10 years after I first saw you. Then I thought, "I've handled this all right, so now I'll retire."

'I found that the reason I had been able to cope was that although I felt lousy nearly every morning and fought my way to work, the moment I became engrossed in work – especially if it was a research project – I felt okay. But sometimes, as soon as I became aware of feeling better, I almost immediately felt awful again. But this is the way it goes, isn't it, doctor? It's an on-and-off affair.'

DOCTOR: 'Yes. Suddenly finding yourself normal acts like a shock, so back come the anxiety and symptoms. You must learn to treat the sudden awareness of normality as one of those flash-moments I have taught you to pass through. Recovery brings many flash-moments that shock.'

PATIENT: 'I can remember right back in my childhood, I had the same experiences. Why was it that when I could play an excellent game of football on important occasions, 10 minutes after playing well, I'd feel suddenly so tired I hardly had the energy to lift one foot off the ground? It was the same when I was going to school. I used to ride 20 miles on horseback each day. Many times I've set out in the morning, most likely in tears, not knowing how I'd face the day and yet, after I settled at school, I'd do a good day's work. I've often wondered, are you born with a predisposition to this sort of thing?'

DOCTOR: 'Some can't summon energy as quickly as others. I remember when I was a student at the university, one senior girl once said to me at breakfast, "I can't bear to look at you,

Essential Help for your Nerves

Weekes! It's indecent to be so energetic so early in the morning!" And yet by night she was firing on all cylinders and I could hardly keep my eyes open. It could be a question of one's particular metabolic rhythm. With you I suspect that the cause was, still is, emotional. You see, you're in your sixties now and I doubt if you would have every reached that age if the cause had been organic. No, I think with you, it has always been emotional.'

PATIENT: 'I think you're right. When my mother's sister was in hospital for a month and I had to visit her every day, I felt better than I had for years. I thought, "This is a crazy business!" I could only figure that I was so busy concentrating on her, I forgot about myself.'

DOCTOR: 'Our thoughts and emotions can be so closely tied that when we establish a pattern of anxious thought, emotional reaction can be triggered so quickly, it seems almost reflexive. Your morning suffering is very much like this; you think, from habit, about feeling tired and then of course, out of habit, you feel tired. If there was something that demanded immediate action, you wouldn't have time to feel fatigued. When you were young, you had only to feel tired on several similar occasions to remember and associate fatigue with that kind of occasion. You established a habit.'

PATIENT: 'I can understand that.'

DOCTOR: 'I remember after a major operation, when I had to return to work after a few weeks and cope with a busy surgery, I would look up the hill I had to climb in the morning and think: "I'll never make it!" Yet later in the day, after walking a few miles between my desk and the examination couch, I felt stronger. If I had spent the day lying about at home thinking about how weak I was, I doubt if I would have recovered so quickly.'

PATIENT: 'It's as I said, with the help of your philosophy and a few tranquillizers occasionally, I got through the last years of my active life. After I retired I was real well for a while. Then I found I was running out of things to do. I still had apprehension about doing certain jobs and when you retire there is a special apprehension, a second lot of challenges to meet!'

DOCTOR: 'When you retire you lose the stimulation of company. There may be too much time to fill in, trying to find jobs, too much time to think about yourself and how you feel.'

PATIENT: 'Making myself do what I know I have to do is the hurdle I have to get over. For example, yesterday I was in this lousy state in the morning thinking, "I've got to play in that wretched game against St Luke's." I thought, "I can't do this!" And then the little voice said, "Well, you've just got to do it! You've just got to have a go, mate!" And sure enough I'd find when I'd get up there and play, it would be okay and when the game's all over, I'd think, "I've been playing this damn match for four hours and I'm feeling good! I should feel exhausted!"'

DOCTOR: 'You know why, of course? During those four hours your mind was on the bowls and not on how you felt. Also, it didn't matter to you how you felt, you knew you had to play on. Not-mattering was the key, as well as thinking of things outside yourself.'

PATIENT: 'There are always odd jobs to cope with and Jerry, my eldest son, usually rings me the night before if I'm going down to help him and says, "Now listen Dad, this is what you've got to bring" and he gives me a list, and then says, "Right. Have you got it all down?" He's a real wag, that one.

'So we set out to go down and I think, "Holy mackerel! I've got to drive down there and it will be a couple of hours going down! That'll be hell!" But by the time I get to the

Harbour Bridge, I've forgotten about worrying and I'm concentrating on driving.'

DOCTOR: 'There is so much habit in your suffering. When you think about a long drive, you imagine doing the whole two hours in one moment of contemplation. Whereas once you start, you do it minute by minute and that's so much easier, especially when your attention is diverted while you drive. When you are sitting contemplating, you concertina the moment into one big obstacle, almost like a concrete wall that has to be got through before you can reach your destination. Action helps tremendously. As I always say: contemplation is the killer. With contemplation you see the whole drive as a very tiring operation and you imagine yourself doing it – the entire drive – during those moments when you are just thinking about it. No wonder it seems tiring!'

FOURTH PATIENT

Recurring Symptoms

PATIENT: 'It's difficult to believe that the symptoms can recur after weeks of peace.'

DOCTOR: 'Yes and they may not come back gently either, even though you are recovering. The contrast between the good you've been feeling and how bad you can suddenly feel seems incredible.'

PATIENT: 'I felt marvellous.'

DOCTOR: 'It is difficult for you to understand and yet the explanation is simple. Recovery from nervous illness is usually fairly slow. You can't quickly forget what you've been through. It's rather like losing through death someone you loved; after a while you can go for weeks without too much suffering and then suddenly the unexpected sight of something belonging to them recalls memories and desolation sweeps again.'

PATIENT: 'That's right. I've had a nasty few days and feel I'll never get better. Desolation? I'll say!'

DOCTOR: 'It's difficult, isn't it, to realize that you are going through a phase of recovery. A strange phase that keeps repeating itself. It's difficult to realize that what will liberate you is simply release from tension through understanding. When you fully understand, it is as if a physical weight is lifted from your chest. You feel freer. Can even think more flexibly.'

PATIENT: 'The most frightening aspect for me is that although there is no reason that I can see, a setback seems to pounce with the force of an elephant. Then I start to wonder: "Am I thinking straight?" Driving over here this afternoon, I was even a bit frightened again and I realized that my thoughts were coming just that fraction slower and this made me apprehensive. Things even looked a little strange.'

DOCTOR: 'You suddenly felt mentally tired in that car. If we were to say that when mentally fresh we function at about 100 per cent of normal, I'd say that you are now functioning at about 75 per cent and that any extra strain, such as driving the car in traffic, although little, can be enough to bring back the symptoms of mental fatigue. Your present reserve of mental energy is low. You may have occasional flashes of feeling 100 per cent – perhaps after a rest or sleep – and these flashes of feeling normal can be very confusing.'

PATIENT: 'Realizing it is only fatigue helps enormously, especially hearing you say it. Fatigue seems to be the key.'

DOCTOR: 'Since your extreme nervous exhaustion, you haven't had a long enough experience of feeling well. You haven't experienced enough to be sure that a setback will always pass.'

PATIENT: 'I have no certainty at all; only your word.'

DOCTOR: 'That's why I say, "Let more time pass."'

PATIENT: 'When I'm working, keeping my train of thought going is very difficult. It's frightening. Sometimes I feel half-witted.'

DOCTOR: 'Don't be afraid of feeling like that. How you feel at that moment is temporary although embarrassing. Remember it is only temporary, and float on. Loosen and accept. Go on quietly, half-witted or not.'

PATIENT: 'Yes and while I am fatigued and sensitized, all the terrible, frightening things going on in the world seem so much more frightening!'

DOCTOR: 'We're all concerned about that, but a sensitized person can feel the concern physically. You know, even announcers make the news seem worse when they hand it out in a doomsday voice. It's a wonder we're not all crazy.'

PATIENT: 'But I shouldn't be frightened like this. It's ridiculous.'

DOCTOR: 'In your present state you are submerged by circumstances. Your control fluctuates; for example, if you have a problem, one day you can see it in perspective – you're on top of it, looking down on it – but the next day, especially if you are tired, it seems on top of you.

'Some days you can think, "Oh yes, I will be able to cope with that!" while the next day you are sure you haven't a hope of coping. You feel as if you have a block in your mind. However, you do cope in spite of the block.'

PATIENT: 'Morning is my worst time. My mind wanders round and round. It's the same every morning. I know I have to get myself used to it. I have to accept that. The thoughts aren't even logical. They come in streams that run in every direction. Again I am apprehensive about recovering.'

DOCTOR: 'As I said, you have no firm foundation for peace yet, no platform from which you can look down on your thoughts. At the moment you are carried away by them like a drowning man in a riptide. Those early morning hours are very difficult to get through, especially when you have to listen to morning sounds you've been hearing for weeks: familiar sounds that bring back the memory of other moments of acute suffering. They seem to drag you back, make you feel you've made no progress. You know?... The dog that starts barking at the same time each morning. Wouldn't you like to shoot it sometimes?'

PATIENT: 'Fortunately we live in a very peaceful spot. I've learned now that the thing to do is to get up and get a drink of something. A glass of hot milk.'

DOCTOR: 'Doing something familiar makes you feel more normal, more real – it breaks the spell.'

PATIENT: 'Yes, but the milk also does seem to settle me.'

DOCTOR: 'There's supposed to be a chemical in milk that helps sleep. However, just going out into a brighter light, being with familiar things helps most, I think. They help you to get strange rambling thoughts into perspective. You can see that they are rambling, that the strangeness is you, going through a special phase in your illness; that is simply born from the way you are feeling at this moment. Don't take any strangeness too seriously at this stage.'

LATER TALK WITH THE SAME PATIENT

HALF BAKED – NOT WITH IT

DOCTOR: 'When you are emerging from nervous illness, feeling good is such a contrast to the way you have so often felt in the past, that the contrast can seem almost like a mild shock. It's the quickness of the body's reaction to the sudden realization of how close suffering is that unbalances. One minute you feel good, the next apprehensive again. You have to learn that such flash-moments are inevitable during recovery and that you have to pass through them again and again. I call going through these flashes being back in the spin-dryer.'

PATIENT: 'Today I've been flicking off the fear quite well, but I had to do it every little while. One flick doesn't do the job!'

DOCTOR: 'Sometimes it seems as if your mind has tentacles that keep clutching and bringing you back to it. You can't understand how you will ever escape them, will ever stop reverting to thinking about yourself. A young man described this well. He said that one night when desperately caught in this trap, a neighbour called and stood talking in the doorway, swinging a lantern. The swinging lantern caught his attention and momentarily he forgot to think inwardly. Suddenly he understood that he could lose this habit of inward thinking just as he could lose any other habit. He could see that it was only a habit. He also saw that it did not matter what he thought; that he could just as well think, "Tick!" as think about himself. He also saw that if he were unafraid of it, any outside interest could claim his attention and the habit itself would be lost. He felt suddenly elated. He had found the way through! He thought, "Flick on! What the heck!" Can you understand this?' (Also discussed on p. 144.)

PATIENT: 'Yes. You mean that when the thoughts flick inward all day, I have to let them flick and know that gradually, as I do this, I will become more interested in doing other things and the habit will go because it won't worry me?'

DOCTOR: 'Yes. Its presence won't matter any more.'

PATIENT: 'That won't be easy to do.'

DOCTOR: 'It's the *only* way.'

PATIENT: 'I get so tired. I can't help sometimes wishing it all to hell!'

DOCTOR: 'Wish that as often as you like, but at the same time understand that it's only memory, habit and fear working together to form this habit. There is no "it" doing this to you; there's just that wretched trio. It's as if your thoughts are caught and made to run in one track. When they've been in that track all day, naturally you despair. But beneath the despair, remember it's only habit, memory, and tenson from fear and fatigue. However, losing this habit is different from losing other habits. You can't think, "I'll stop!" and then stop (for instance, like stopping smoking). You must let it come and learn to make it part of your ordinary thinking and not think of it as forbidden territory – something you must not think.'

PATIENT: 'When I talk to you I understand and feel courage and am sure I will be able to do it. But as well as losing that habit, what worries me is the feeling of being half-baked, not "with it".'

DOCTOR: 'That's mental fatigue. This is the devil, isn't it? And you're going through a lot of it because of your constant anxiety about it and the kind of brainwork you do. Don't think, "I've got to find a way out of all this!" You haven't. Your body, your mind, will find a way if you simply remember acceptance. Accept and let your body and mind do the rest. There is no mystery. Accept whatever happens at the moment, even though you may think it's driving you crackers.'

PATIENT: 'That's just what's been making me so fearful – the thought that I'm going mad!'

DOCTOR: 'And when fearful, you become especially tense and that's when ideas really stick and that's when you think you're going mad. You've tried to live with so much, to conquer so much.'

PATIENT: 'Two weeks ago I was free! What's happened now to take me back into it all again?'

DOCTOR: 'Don't look back. You must look forward. You are still very vulnerable to repeats of "it", please accept that. But of course, then comes that strange experience that when you do relax and are free, you think, "I hope I don't have to go back into that again!" You tense at this very thought and of course, you can then be so easily drawn into thinking inwardly once more. But that's part of getting better. Take the whole lot and think, "What will be will be!" Don't try to direct. Submit. Hang the lot! And take what comes!'

PATIENT: 'I'm doing that 95 per cent of the time, but I slip back on the other 5 per cent.'

DOCTOR: 'You think you've slipped back but all you've done is to slip once more into the wrong groove. Thoughts quickly become grooved. Your thoughts repeat themselves like a needle stuck in the groove of a record. You think there is no way out. There is. Accept the groove always as part of your ordinary thinking. *Stay in the groove willingly.*'

PATIENT: 'Here we go again!'

He went very well indeed.

CHAPTER 7

❦

Talk Given at National Phobia Conference

Talk given as guest speaker at the fourth National Phobia Conference sponsored by the Phobia Society of America and Phobia Clinic, White Plains Hospital Medical Center, New York, 7 May 1983

As we all know, there are many different ways of treating nervous illness, I am speaking now of anxiety states with, or without, obsessions, phobias.

I recently read a book in which the author described most of the common methods of treatment of nervous illness used today. While they seemed different, they each claimed a good record of success. Whatever the treatment, in my opinion, success will depend on the sufferer's attitude to it.

If he is convinced that it will help him, the chances are it will: you know the saying, 'Nothing is but thinking makes it so.' However, in my opinion, a treatment based mainly on belief in it is in danger of working only temporarily. While ever the person treated continues to believe that it will work, he's probably safe, but let him begin to doubt and he's in for trouble. Let him begin to doubt any outside crutch on which he depends and he's in danger.

For recovery, the sufferer must have, deep within himself, a special voice that says during any setback or dark moment, 'It's all right; you've been here before. You know the way out. You can do it again. It works, you know it works!' That voice speaks with authority and brings comfort only when it has been earned by the sufferer himself and it can be earned only by making the symptoms and experiences that torture *no longer matter*. NO LONGER MATTERING IS THE KEY. It is not a question of some method of treatment spiriting misery away, anaesthetizing it. It is a question of the symptoms, the experiences, no longer mattering.

The necessity for the sufferer himself to earn the inner voice of assurance does not exclude outside help; for example, by giving understanding and direction and if possible by alleviating difficult, stressful circumstances.

The person alone all day with no programme of recovery to follow, no special interesting work to do, who has somehow to fill each hour (the exhausted housewife struggling to cope with the work, perhaps with a couple of children dragging at her skirt), the person who thinks himself too ill and weary to work, and who is ill and weary with adrenal glands depleted by too intense and too frequent stress – what a mountain such people have to climb to earn that inner voice, especially if panic and other symptoms come by merely thinking about them.

These people's minds are all geared ready to thwart; ready at every turn to put up a barricade. The mind will remember and remind, mock, tantalize, never leaving the body alone. It will twist, turn, spiral, cavort – always turning inward, inward, inward, clinging with tentacles of glue.

And yet all through this turmoil, the right comforting voice is there to be discovered. However, the sufferer needs to be shown how to make this discovery, how to make his torture no longer matter. It is not enough to simply have it subdued. Balance must be struck between the sufferer doing the work by himself and being helped. So the question is: What outside help should be given? First, let us consider tranquillization.

A while ago, I read in a London newspaper an article by a journalist who said she had been agoraphobic for many years, but could now go anywhere simply by taking a certain tablet three times a day. She gave the name of the pill; said she'd tried all the others and that none had worked as well as this one.

'And now,' said she, 'all I have to do is come off that little pill!' Only that! She had no idea that she was announcing that she had left her future in the hands of chance. She had left it to chance, because so much would depend on what she thought on the very day when she first went without her pills. I notice she wrote the article first.

If, on that special day, she thought, 'Well, all is well ... I can go anywhere now. I don't need the pill. The pill's not important any longer; so I can forget about it!' – if she thought that way and did forget about the pill, all could be well – temporarily. I say temporarily, because if stress – similar to the stress that had originally brought her symptoms – returned, or if she simply thought of panic and panicked (particularly in some awkward situation) I wonder how long it would be before she reached for a pill? I don't really wonder; I know. It wouldn't be very long. And when she succumbed, how long before her inner voice said, 'You'll probably always need that pill, you know!' And that would be her master's voice speaking. The pill would be the master now.

And the voice could go on and say, 'And what will you do if it doesn't work this time! What will you do then?' I leave you to use your imagination about that one. (Also discussed on p. 28.)

There is another kind of outside help; the kind used by quite a few self-help groups that teach members to go as far as they can without panicking and then if they feel panic, to come back and try again another day, until they can do that particular journey comfortably – without panicking.

But what will the inner voice say if, having got used to all those places, one day, when out, a member of that group – perhaps tired, perhaps sensitized by some worry, or perhaps simply remembering how he used to panic – what if he panics again! What does his little voice say then? It has a heyday.

One man in Canada belonged to a group of agoraphobic people who worked this way. He felt so far recovered that he was able to travel into the United States and managed very well. I believe he went as far as Las Vegas and did not panic.

The day after he returned home he went down to the bank to draw some money. The same old bank, the same teller with the thick-lensed glasses, even the same bankbook with the torn corner, and as he handed the bankbook to the teller he stood on the exact spot where he had so often panicked before. Of course, memory smote, and on came panic and *it was a smasher!* It beat all records, because with it came anguish and despair – above all, despair. From then on, he wasn't even back in square one; he was back in square minus-one. And his inner voice shouted, 'What are you going to do now? If, after all those months of getting-used-to, after all those weeks of successful travelling in the United States, if after all that, you can't even go to your bank without panicking, what *are* you going to do now?' (Also discussed on p. 27.)

Then there is the person who gets help from a special doctor and who uses the doctor as a more or less permanent crutch. What happens if that doctor leaves the district? And the sufferer has to depend on himself? (He doesn't like the other doctors in the town much and they're not too keen on him.) What does his inner voice say? Well, it says the same old, 'What are you going to do now? You're really lost this time, brother!'

That doctor had been very kind and thoughtful but he had been no real help. He'd been a crutch for too long.

There is only one way to cure and that is for the therapist to help his patient develop an inner voice that says in a crisis, 'Go on, through. You've done it before. It works. You know it works. On, through!' An inner voice that is followed by a feeling of inner strength. *A real physical feeling*. Almost as if a piece of iron rod takes the place of quivering jelly.

Some of you are, I know, sceptical of my using the word cure, especially if I had said permanent cure. I am aware that many therapists believe there is no permanent cure for nervous illness. When I was on radio some years ago in New York with a physician and a psychiatrist, the psychiatrist corrected me when I used the word cure and said, 'You mean remission, don't you, Dr Weekes? We never speak of curing nervous illness!' I told her that I had cured far too many nervously ill people to be afraid to use the word.

I suppose were we to say that if a person saw a murder committed before his eyes, there would be no hope of his completely forgetting it, and we would be right. I think that perhaps that is what some therapists mean when they say nervous illness cannot be cured, only relieved. They believe that memory will always return and that the nerves of a once nervously ill person may respond to memory with such intensity because of their past experience, that the poor devil is doomed. I think maybe that's what they mean. Also I suspect that some therapists, who deny cure of nervous illness, may think 'Once a weakling, always a weakling.' Maybe.

Of course, memory is always capable of recalling nervous symptoms and what a heyday an anxious inner voice has then.

It says, 'It's all back again! Every lock, stock and barrel. Every member of the family! We're all here. What are you going to do now? You'll never recover now, you know!' What power the wrong voice holds. But if the right earned voice is there it will come to the rescue and say, 'You've been here before, you know the way!' Then, in spite of being possibly shocked and temporarily thrown off balance, the owner of that inner voice does know what to do and gradually does it.

And that's what I mean by cure: having the right inner voice to support and lead through setbacks, through flash-moments of despair, through bewilderment. That is cure. I don't mean that the once-nervously-ill person will always be at peace, will not have setbacks. Of course he may; surely he's entitled to be human. I mean that for a person to be cured, he must be able to take setbacks as they come (and they may come unexpectedly 30 years or more after the original illness); must take the setback directed by an inner voice that is the real tranquillizer. This is my meaning of cure.

And after each setback that inner voice is strengthened and what is more, each setback successfully navigated by that voice reinforces confidence, self esteem. Can you see how important, almost essential, setbacks are when the right inner voice is being developed to be the guide?

I suppose it's a lucky person who goes through life without being nervously ill. But I wonder. A person who has been nervously ill has widened his understanding, his power to appreciate, to feel compassion, even to enjoy.

But of course he has to carry the scar of memory. You know the saying, 'Where ignorance is bliss, 'tis folly to be wise.' But if the sufferer has developed the strong, right inner voice, there is not so much folly for him in being wise.

But without the right voice, all is left to chance and that's very chancey. Also, the person, who has been 'cured' (and I put 'cured' in quotes) by chance, by luck, by some outside crutch on which he continues to depend, can know only the peace of ignorance and that's no peace at all. It is only a temporary quietness. As long as his luck holds, he's probably okay. But luck has a habit of changing. It's a fool who trusts his life to luck and we are talking about people's lives.

So I believe, in the work I have done, I have tried to show the patient how to develop the right inner voice. The person who recovers using the four concepts that I teach – facing, accepting, floating, and letting time pass – has done so by *going through hell the right way* and so has developed that right inner voice.

But in doing so, he has to put his head on the block: has to put himself into stressful situations that he otherwise would have avoided. And that's where he often falters, even sometimes fails. However, I teach him to know that peace lies on the other side of panic, on the other side of failure, never on this side.

There is a clinic in Toronto, Canada, specializing in treating nervous illness and the superintendent wrote to me and asked permission to use phrases from one of my books. He said he had these printed on ballpoint pens which he gave to patients. One of the phrases chosen was: 'Recovery lies in the places and experiences you fear.' And that in my opinion is exactly right. I teach my patients never to be put off by the places and experiences they fear. These are their salvation.

The person who ventures into these places and experiences will of course sensitize himself more than if he avoided them; so I come again to the question of tranquillization.

For some people I prescribe temporary tranquillizaton but of course, I tailor the dose to the person. I always bear in mind that to earn the right kind of inner voice, the sufferer must go through his experiences acutely enough to learn that facing, accepting, and floating do the real work. He would never know this if he were continuously tranquillized. As I say, the question of tranquillization is a delicate one and must be tailored to the individual.

There are people who can, and prefer to, go through the greatest hell without tranquillizers; however, the majority want, and need, to be helped with tranquillizers during the most severe stages of their illness.

Nervous illness is so very tiring. There is not only muscular, emotional, and mental fatigue, there is also a kind of fatigue of the spirit, when the will to survive falters. I have found that when people reach this stage, to sedate and let them sleep even for a few hours can make all the difference. It can refresh enough for them to find courage and strength to go on once more.

In my opinion, this is one of the main uses of tranquillizers – to relieve fatigue and also to take the sharp edge off suffering, when suffering becomes almost too great for a body to bear.

I say almost, because there are those who can and do bear it. However, we should never demand this unreasonably from our patients. As I say, tranquillization must be temporary and tailored to the individual.

So I leave you all with a suggestion: those of you treating nervous illness should find out what the inner voice of your patients is saying. In my opinion, when we think we have cured a patient but have not helped him earn the right inner voice, we have not cured at all, whatever method used.

If some of you suffer from nervous illness; find out what your inner voice is saying. Be honest about it. Face it. If it brings no reassurances, find a voice that does – by facing, accepting, floating and letting time pass. And remember, when we learn to walk and live *with* fear, we eventually walk and live *without* fear.

BOOK 2

❦

PEACE
from
NERVOUS
SUFFERING

Preface

Peace From Nervous Suffering is offered as a treatment for nervous illness, not merely as reading. The nervously disturbed person is often so tired and confused, he finds concentrating and remembering difficult; therefore I have written this with as much emphasis – repetition, even italics – as I thought helpful.

In my earlier book, *Self-Help For Your Nerves*, I talked about the commonest kind of nervous illness – the anxiety state (often called nervous breakdown). In this book, while I offer additional special help to those suffering the anxiety state in general, I offer especial help to those whose illness is dominated by a particular fear – agoraphobia. Agoraphobia is a fear of leaving the safety of the home; of travelling alone – even as far as the corner of the street to post a letter. It includes fear of wide open spaces, as well as fear of being in crowded places – the school hall, restaurant, even church.

To my knowledge, this is the first book written by a doctor directly to sufferers from this crippling illness. Indeed, other than treatises on agoraphobia written for medical journals, or mention of it in books on fears or phobias, this is the first book written mainly on agoraphobia itself.

It is estimated that more than 300,000 people suffer from agoraphobia in Britain alone. The number is probably far greater, as so many sufferers do not seek help for their illness; many even hide it. Although so widespread, agoraphobia has only recently been recognized by doctors generally. However, it is arousing much interest in Britain and America today, and the future promises improved understanding and treatment for many people who, so far, have thought themselves alone, unnoticed, even unique in their illness.

During 1968–1970 I wrote eight quarterly journals for 1,300 sufferers from nervous illness – the majority with agoraphobia – in the British Isles, the United States of America, Canada, Australia, New Zealand, South Africa, Hong Kong, India and recently Japan. These journals are already well known, but this is their first printing in book form.

Claire Weekes
London
January 1971

Contents

The Housebound Housewife,
the Citybound Executive

⋏

CHAPTER 1

Sensitization:
The Simple Cause of so much
Nervous Illness

If nervous suffering has led you to this book, you may have picked it up with both hope and doubt.

You have possibly tried so hard to recover in the past and have – as you think – let yourself down so often, you may hesitate to trust yourself to try again. Perhaps you have been ill so long, you suspect you are beyond help.

Small wonder doubt is mixed with hope. And yet, I assure you, however often you may have failed in the past, however long you may have suffered, you can recover.

Perhaps, like so many of my nervously ill patients, you have no personality defect making or keeping you ill; indeed, you may have no particular problem. Many of my patients were happy in their home life and at work, until they became ill. They then became afraid of the state they were in, *of the way they felt,* afraid not only of what was happening at the time but also of what they feared might yet be in store. Without realizing it their nerves had tricked them; duped them.

EVERY SHADE OF EVERY TRICK

Through the years, I have seen every shade of every trick my patients' nerves have played upon them, and because they were so easily, so unwittingly led into nervous illness in this way, I want to open your eyes to the way your nerves could now be tricking you.

After explanation, some people have said, 'If I had known that a year ago, Doctor!' Some have even said, 'If I had only known that forty years ago!' – the best part of a lifetime sacrificed through ignorance of something we should all know as well as we know our own name. We should know there are three special pitfalls that can lead into nervous illness, and above all, we should know how to cope with them.

The three pitfalls are *sensitization*, *bewilderment* and *fear*. Sensitization is a state in which nerves are conditioned to react to stress in an exaggerated way; that is, they bring unusually intense feelings when under stress, and at times with alarming swiftness.

There is no mystery about sensitization. Most of us have surely felt it in a mild way at the end of a tense day's work, when nerves feel on edge and little things upset us too much. Constant tension has alerted our nerves to react in a mildly exaggerated way. It is not pleasant, we do not like it, but we do not let it distract us too much.

Severe sensitization, on the other hand, can be very upsetting. A severely sensitized person may feel his heart constantly beating quickly, thumping, or 'skipping' beats; he may have recurring attacks of palpitations; may feel his stomach 'churn' – especially on waking in the morning, or after an afternoon nap; his hands may tremble, sweat; he may have difficulty expanding his chest sufficiently to take in a deep breath and may 'gasp and gulp for air (in the words of one woman), thinking he is suffocating, even about to die. He may suffer from weak 'turns' and may complain of a lump in his throat which, he says, interferes with swallowing solid food. He has headaches; a feeling of weight pressing on top of the head, an 'iron band' around the head; giddiness; a feeling of lurching, swaying, or light-headedness. Most alarming of all, panic may come so swiftly, so easily, that even the slight shock of missing a step in the dark, a cold blast of wind, or a slamming door, may bring a whipping lash of panic in a severely sensitized person. More bewildering still, panic may seem to come for no apparent reason.

Although these are no more than the usual symptoms of stress exaggerated by sensitization, the exaggeration is so upsetting, so baffling, the sufferer rarely recognizes them as stress symptoms. He thinks they are unique to him, that no one could have suffered this way before.

SUDDEN SENSITIZATION

One does not need to be a special type of person to become severely sensitized. Severe sensitization can be suddenly, unexpectedly thrust upon any one of us at any time. Hence the need to understand it and know how to cope with it. It may follow the stress of physical shock to our nerves, such as an accident, an exhausting surgical operation, a difficult confinement, a severe haemorrhage, and so on.

Some nervous reaction is expected in any of these situations. However, occasionally it can be unexpectedly severe. For example, when severe sensitization follows a surgical operation, post-operative routines – such as the simple finger-prick for a blood-count, or dressing a wound – can almost reduce their victim to tears. Any frustration, perhaps no more than waiting for the doctor to arrive, may bring intense agitation and make nerves feel so taut, that a sudden noise jars painfully. Also, panic can follow the slightest anxious thought.

A retiring nursing sister who had been for years in charge of a surgical ward said recently, 'If I had known more about sensitization when I was nursing, what a difference it would have made to the extra understanding I could have given my patients and what added satisfaction I could have had from my work.' At that time she was sensitized herself.

GRADUAL SENSITIZATION

Of course, severe sensitization can come more slowly. It may gradually accompany continuous domestic stress; too strenuous dieting; any debilitating illness; anaemia – anything which puts nerves under stress for a considerable time. The strain need not necessarily be unhappy; an actor constantly alerted to give his best performance can become quite severely sensitized, especially if he neglects sleep and food.

ALWAYS THE SAME EFFECT

Since the symptoms of sensitization are the symptoms of stress, they conform to the usual pattern of stress and this pattern is set, limited, because nerves under stress always release the same chemicals to act on the same organs and always produce the same results. It comforts a sufferer to learn that the pattern of his suffering is limited and that he has probably already experienced the severest symptoms his nerves can bring. I have seen

Essential Help for Your Nerves

this information alone cure some people in an anxiety state. Because their body had brought them so many surprises in the past, and had – as they thought – let them down so badly, they had been constantly worried about what further surprises the future might hold.

'ONLY NERVES'

When we say someone is suffering from nerves, we do not only mean that nerves are stimulated to bring certain symptoms; we also imply that the nerves have 'gone wrong', are somehow to blame. Actually, they are responding faithfully and physiologically to the messages sent to them. To be cured, it is essential to understand this, and to do so we should know how our nerves normally function. Although I described this in detail in my earlier book, *Self Help for Your Nerves*, it is necessary to repeat it, at least briefly, here.

Our nervous system consists of two parts, voluntary and involuntary. By means of our voluntary nerves we move our muscles (hence, our body) more or less as we wish. These nerves obey our direct command – so they are called voluntary.

The involuntary nerves help our glands to control the functioning of our organs – heart, lungs, bowels, and so on. Unlike the voluntary nerves, these nerves are not under our direct control - hence the term involuntary.

The involuntary nerves themselves consist of two types, sympathetic and parasympathetic. In a peaceful body sympathetic and parasympathetic nerves hold each other in check. However, if we are emotional – afraid, angry, excited, agitated – one dominates the other (usually the sympathetic dominates the parasympathetic) and we are aware of certain organs functioning; we may feel our heart race, pound; may breathe quickly; our hands may sweat, and so on. Sympathetic nerves react this way mainly by means of a chemical called adrenalin which is released at the nerve-endings in the organs concerned.

Normally, when afraid, we accept our racing heart, rapid breathing, even the spasm of fear in our 'middle' because we know that when the cause of fear goes these reactions will also pass. Our feelings calm because we change our mood. *Changing mood (attitude) is the only conscious control, other than medication, we have over our involuntary nerves and so over our symptoms of stress.*

I emphasize this because understanding it is of paramount importance in understanding recovery from so much nervous illness.

WHAT KEEPS A PERSON SENSITIZED?

Now I come to a point I wish to highlight: *the symptoms of so much nervous illness are no more than the symptoms of stress exaggerated by severe sensitization.* One might well ask: Is there a difference between severe sensitization and nervous illness? If so, when do we say someone is merely sensitized and when nervously ill? And how does one pass from sensitization to nervous illness?

We say a person is nervously ill, and not merely sensitized, when sensitization upsets him so much that it interferes with his way of life. Someone who has never been sensitized, or nervously ill, might well then ask: What keeps a person sensitized long enough for this to happen? And this is a good question, because it brings us face to face with those other two culprits, bewilderment and fear. Bewilderment and fear keep sensitization alive. Bewilderment acts by placing a sensitized person constantly under the strain of asking himself: 'What is wrong with me?

Why am I like this?' The more he struggles to be the person he was, the more exasperation, tension, he adds and, of course, the more stress. His failure to find a way out of this maze makes him feel incapable of coping not only with present difficulties but also with whatever future course his illness might take, and he vaguely sees himself being 'taken away somewhere'.

While he feels, in his bewilderment, that he cannot direct his thoughts and actions adequately, he stands especially vulnerable to, and defenceless before, fear, which can overwhelm him before he has time to reason with it. It is the stress of bewilderment and fear continually being added to the stress of the original sensitization that keeps this sensitization alive, keeps the symptoms of stress so severe. The sensitized person puts himself in a cycle of fear-adrenalin-fear. In other words, his fear of the state he is in produces the adrenalin and other stress hormones, which continue to excite his nerves to produce the very symptoms he fears. The fear-adrenalin-fear cycle is also called an anxiety state.

As explained in my earlier book, the majority of people who have come to me for help have had no subconscious cause either beginning their illness or keeping them ill. Indeed many had no particular problem, other than finding the way to recovery, or trying to meet responsibilities which, because of illness, seemed beyond them. They had been tricked into illness by those three bogeys: sensitization, bewilderment and fear.

THE HABIT OF FEAR

In my opinion, too much time is spent and too much unnecessary suffering caused today by frequently searching for deep-seated causes for nervous illness, when so often none exists. It is not enough to be told that such and such happened when one was young and that is why one is so nervous now. Whatever may have originally caused the illness – and in my opinion, it is not so often a childhood cause as many believe – *present sensitization remains*. The habit of fear is the important thing now. *This must be cured*.

A woman from America wrote, 'I saw a doctor four years ago, but out of sheer frustration of his continually rehashing the past, I quit. All I seemed to hear was that my mother left me to the maids and my father didn't love me either. I have been told over and over again that lack of love has caused my acute phobias, but never how to handle the fears themselves, especially the fear of leaving home alone. I have repeatedly asked for help to deal with today, with the acute and constant fears and awful physical feelings I have. It seems that all I've been given to live with is "but if" and "if only".'

This is not an isolated cry; it comes from many.

AT THE BACK OF THE HALL, 'JUST IN CASE'

The sensitized person is afraid of so much. He will sit at the back of the hall at the school meeting; near the door in the restaurant; on the aisle in the cinema; at the end of the last row of pews in church, so that he can slip out unnoticed if, as he thinks, his fears grow beyond him. He always leaves a way open for quick retreat, 'just in case'. A nervously ill woman cancels her appointment with the hairdresser or dentist again and again. Retreat is not quick enough from that chair!

In my opinion, until the importance of straightforward sensitization is recognized as a possible cause of nervous illness, our present rate of cure will not improve as much as it otherwise would. I stress again that so much nervous illness has no deep-seated cause and is no more than severe sensitization kept alive by bewilderment and fear.

IF YOU WISH TO RECOVER, YOU CAN

The nervously disturbed person is forever questioning not only himself but others, and too often the answers are so unsatisfactory that he loses hope of ever finding the explanation he craves, especially if he has been ill for a long time. Should you suffer in this way, you need a full explanation of what is happening to you, as well as a definite programme for recovery. These are given in this book.

I stress: *however long you may have suffered from nervous illness, if you wish to recover, you can.* The main difference between a person ill for many years and someone ill for a short time is that the one who has suffered for long has had much more time to collect disturbing memories, especially the memory of much defeat, so that he despairs easily. But the years of suffering have not so affected him physically that he cannot recover now.

However long you have been ill, your body is waiting to recover in the same way as the body of a person who has been ill for only a short time; the same processes of recovery are waiting to work as well for you as for anyone else. It is important to understand this, because your illness is an illness of how you think. *It is very much an illness of your attitude to fear.* You may think yours is an illness of how you feel – it certainly seems like that – but how you feel depends on how you think. And this is good, because thoughts that are keeping you ill can be changed. That is, your approach to your illness can be changed.

Now do not despair when you read this. I know how easily you despair; how acutely you feel at the mercy of some 'thing' propelling you against your will, and how impossible it may seem at this moment to even imagine changing your approach to your illness. But it is my work to help you, to show you the way. Take heart.

When I see a person who has been nervously ill for a long time, I do not think of him, or her, as hopelessly, chronically ill; neither do I see a coward. I see a suffering, bewildered, and often brave person, who has possibly not had adequate explanation of his illness, adequate help. So many people have been cured at last after being ill for many years that I, as a doctor, am rarely deterred by a patient's history of long illness. So, do not be discouraged if your illness has been called 'chronic'. I assure you, once again, if you want to recover and are willing to follow the advice in this book, you can recover.

Of course, many people have special problems which started their illness and are now helping to keep them ill and naturally these must be met before complete recovery is possible. Chapter 5 is on solving the apparently insoluble problem.

Also, there is more to nervous illness than the physical symptoms mentioned – panic, palpitations, weak turns and so on. Fear, and its resulting tension, can bring some most disconcerting experiences. In later chapters I briefly discuss such experiences as inability to make decisions; suggestibility; loss of confidence; feelings of unreality and personality disintegration; obsession; depression. These are discussed more fully in my earlier book.

In the next chapter I examine in detail perhaps the most crippling of all fears that make part of an anxiety state – fear of leaving the safety of home (agoraphobia).

CHAPTER 2

⚘

Fear of Leaving the Safety of Home (Agoraphobia)

Most people have heard of claustrophobia – fear of enclosed places – but few have heard of agoraphobia, a much more incapacitating fear. Agoraphobia literally means 'fear of the market place'; in medical practice it means fear of leaving the safety of home, either alone or in the company of others. It includes fear of entering shops, travelling in a car or public vehicle, and sometimes even fear of walking as far as the end of the street.

Until recently, agoraphobia was not recognized; even some doctors had not heard of the term. Four years ago, I accompanied a patient to see an ophthalmic surgeon of many years' experience. I explained to him that the patient suffered from agoraphobia and mentioned the possible temporary effect of the tension on her vision. He listened politely, but when we were leaving, said, 'I don't believe in this illness you call agoraphobia. It doesn't exist!'

Since then there has been much publicity in England about the agoraphobic housebound housewife in newspapers and magazines, and on radio and television, and I doubt if that surgeon would say the same today.

It is possible this particular phase of nervous illness received so little attention in the past because an agoraphobic person often feels too selfconscious about his fears to discuss them even with a doctor. It is not easy for a woman to confess, especially to a man who she thinks may be unbelieving (as was that surgeon), that she is afraid to go to the supermarket alone and must either take a child with her for protection, or send the child to do the shopping. It is just as difficult for a man to explain that he prefers to stay in a subordinate position at work because he cannot face taking a higher appointment which would mean travelling from city to city while he finds it so difficult to leave his own town. This fear is not only difficult to explain to others but also difficult for the sufferers themselves to understand. Most of them used not to be like this, and look back now in amazement at how freely they could once travel. This is why they think their illness is peculiar, something to be ashamed of, and why they are so surprised when they learn that many sensible, even notable, people suffer just as they do.

After I have spoken about agoraphobia on radio or television, the studio switchboard is frequently jammed with incoming calls from people who have heard themselves and their fears described for the first time. Acknowledgement that the origin of their illness could be simple, together with the detailed description of how they feel – especially recognition of the importance of their fear of fear – is the reassurance they had been wanting for so long and had despaired of finding. So often, the complicated reasons for their illness previously given to those who had sought help had confused and disheartened more than helped.

One might surely ask how such a strange condition arises, because it seems so extraordinarily childish to be unable to walk as far as the end of the road to post a letter.

So often agoraphobia begins understandably enough. In the first place, it should be understood that the sufferer does not really think some particular place holds a special danger for him; that something there will harm him. He is afraid of how he will *react* when in a certain situation. He has become so sensitively aware of what happens within himself at the slightest stress – of how he panics, feels weak, giddy, and so on – that he lives in fear of these feelings coming where he thinks he will be unable to cope with them, and where he may consequently make a fool of himself in front of others. So, the housewife clings to her home, and the executive to his own home-town. Each clings to his safety zone.

This is why the nervous person sits at the back of the school meeting, on the aisle at the cinema, near the door in the restaurant – so that he can slip out quickly and unnoticed if he feels one of his turns coming. He especially dreads being in an aeroplane, a train, or any vehicle he cannot stop and leave at will.

The interest aroused in agoraphobia today has led to surveys being made – principally in the British Isles – of groups of agoraphobic sufferers with special regard to cause and results of treatment. In my experience, the cause in most people has been easy to find. So often agoraphobia begins with an unexpected attack of weakness – a feeling of collapse – while out. Frequently it has followed a sudden, unaccountable attack of severe panic. The basic cause of these attacks has usually been fatigue, or some other form of stress, following a variety of experiences, some of which I have already mentioned – difficult confinement, debilitating illness, and so on. Occasionally there is no obvious reason and, happily, I have rarely found disclosing an original cause of agoraphobia essential for cure.

It will surely be appreciated how easily a housewife can be frightened by an attack of palpitations and then afraid to venture far from home for fear of having a 'heart attack' while out. Anything unusual to do with the heart is upsetting, and a sudden attack of palpitations can be alarming, especially if it comes when alone and away from home. If the sufferer has more than one attack, she may be convinced there is something radically wrong with her heart. If she goes immediately to a doctor who reassures her that the trouble is 'only nerves' and helps her to become reconciled to perhaps having an occasional attack until her health improves, all will be well. However, if she does not accept his reassurance, she may be constantly worried about her heart – especially if she has further attacks – and may be especially afraid the palpitations will come where she cannot get help readily. Hence a growing reluctance to move far from home.

HIS WIFE WENT EVERYWHERE WITH HIM

A lecturer, afraid of having an attack of palpitations while speaking before an audience, gradually lost so much confidence that he would not speak unless his wife was present. This is not as childish as it sounds, because he was most likely to have an attack when apprehensive and he was most apprehensive while lecturing. His wife's presence gave him a feeling of support which allayed his fear.

If a housewife, afraid of a heart attack (as she wrongly diagnoses palpitations), or of a weak turn, or of panic, manages to walk as far as the supermarket, how natural, when faced with waiting in the queue at the check-out, to be suddenly smitten with the thought, 'What if I had a turn now?' Fear and tension can quickly agitate a sensitized person and the feeling of vulnerability that comes with agitation will soon convince her that her symptoms could build up into one of her spells. Hence her eventual decision to avoid the supermarket, or to find someone to shop with her.

WOMAN RATHER THAN MAN

I speak now of woman rather than man, because more women than men suffer from agoraphobia. A woman's life at home lends itself to the development of agoraphobia. However, there are agoraphobic men and they, as mentioned earlier, while accustomed to leaving the house daily, usually show their illness by refusing to leave their own town. Many a deputy chief would be chief today were he not afraid of the travelling involved by seniority. I call this the citybound executive syndrome.

Symptoms are no respecter of sex. A nervously ill man complains of the same symptoms as a nervous woman – palpitations, weak turns, giddiness, trembling, panic. These symptoms are not as 'feminine' as one has been conditioned to think. They are the symptoms of stress and therefore experienced by men and women alike.

Weak spells are just as upsetting as palpitations. If the sufferer panics while out because of having a weak spell, she may feel so exhausted she is sure she can go no further and must return home. But how quickly those weak legs move when once headed towards the house. If, instead of returning home, she tries to fight her way forward, or by grim determination stays in the supermarket (or any other place), mounting tension may so stiffen her muscles, she may feel 'seized up' and stand 'paralysed', holding on to the nearest support, unable – as she thinks – to move. She especially dreads a big emporium, where the crowd, heat, noise, and the absence of a place to sit seem to invite that faint feeling.

THE PAVEMENT SEEMS TO HEAVE

Giddiness is especially dreaded and the sufferer is not so easily convinced that such a disturbing physical sensation can be caused by nerves. One woman said, 'when I am overtired, I get giddy and I've still got to convince myself the giddiness is only fatigue, because when I am tired it's hard to convince myself of anything.'

The thought of brain tumour may haunt her. Even if finally persuaded that nerves are the culprit, she finds walking down the street difficult while the pavement seems to heave; the shops to topple. Nor is it easy to stay in the supermarket while the goods on the shelves seem to sway.

In addition, tension may affect her sight, so that, from time to time, objects appear blurred and the distant view covered with a shimmering haze.

Surely it is not difficult to understand how this woman, having these experiences, gradually prefers to stay at home, or take someone – even a child – to shop with her. If she takes a child, it may not be long before she becomes afraid the child will notice her peculiarities and see her 'like this'; so she may postpone shopping until her husband can accompany her.

EXPOSING A CHILDHOOD CAUSE RARELY HELPS

An important part of treatment lies in showing a sensitized woman, or man, how to cope with the exaggerated symptoms of stress, particularly panic, so that they gradually desensitize themselves, and, if agoraphobic, are no longer afraid to be alone, travel alone, be surrounded by people, or take the strain of waiting in a queue. As I said earlier, finding a childhood cause for present illness may be interesting, but it rarely helps cope with the present condition, especially if the sufferer has been ill a long time.

A happily married woman who suffered for years from agoraphobia was told by an analyst that her reluctance to go out alone was based on a subconscious fear of becoming a prostitute. This woman had begun to have faint spells while driving a munition waggon during the Second World War and naturally lost confidence in driving alone. The cause of her turns was probably fatigue. She had certainly not had enough rest or food. However, it was obvious from her history that the attacks she had later, during the years that followed, were induced by memory and fear of having a turn where she could not get help, or where one would be humiliating or dangerous – in a crowd, driving a car and so on. The orbit within which she could move gradually became so restricted that she could finally drive only a few miles from home, could not enter a big store alone, and could go on holiday only if accompanied by a doctor, there and back. Naturally, she and the family took few holidays.

She was finally taught by explanation and encouragement how to cope with her fears. Part of her story, written by herself, is in Journal 8 (Chapter 16).

CONFIDENT ON MONDAY; DEFEATED ON TUESDAY

So much depends on a doctor's ability to explain why, when the patient is feeling better, setback can come for no special reason – at least none that he can see – and be so immediately devastating, as if no progress had been made; to explain why symptoms thought forgotten can return so acutely after months of absence;

why all the symptoms can appear, one after the other; why panic can come 'out of the blue'; why such demoralizing exhaustion can so rapidly follow stress; why, despite the right attitude, sensitization may sometimes linger on for such an unexpectedly long time; why, on returning home after being especially successful, it may seem as if no success had been achieved and why going out the next day can be as difficult as ever. The 'whys' seem countless.

Unless a doctor has the necessary understanding, it is not surprising if his attitude towards curing agoraphobia may be pessimistic. An agoraphobic woman wrote about herself and fellow sufferers, 'If unmarried, we may be patted on the back and told we will be better when married; if married, that having a child will fix us; if middle-aged, that it's "the change"!'

TO BE AFRAID IS SO HUMAN

During interviews on radio and television, I have been surprised at the intensity with which some of my colleagues have defended their belief that the anxiety state, including agoraphobia, is due either to some deep-seated cause, often thought to be subconscious, or to some character inadequacy and that the illness can be cured only if these causes are found and treated.

But severe sensitization, as already pointed out, can come to any one of us at any time, and to be bewildered by and afraid of its acute and baffling symptoms is so human, so natural, it is difficult to understand why the many people who respond this way should be thought inadequate, or different; or why finding some deep-seated cause should be thought essential. Sudden severe sensitization can be shocking, confidence can be quickly shattered, and one does not have to be a dependent type – as I have sometimes heard these sufferers described – to be so affected. If some nervously ill doctors can, with their medical training, fail to understand sensitization, or know how to cope with its effects on themselves (and I have seen this), why should a layman be expected *as a matter of course* to be wise enough to do so, and to be philosophical about it into the bargain?

Fear is one of the strongest, most disagreeable emotions we know. Is it inconceivable that one could be afraid of it for its own sake? Must there always be a cause of fear other than fear of fear? Why cannot fear of fear, when it flashes almost electrically – as it can in a sensitized person – be a cause in itself? It is, you know.

Far from being dependent types, many nervously ill people, although unable to understand what is happening, show great courage and independence fighting their fears, often with little help or sympathy from their families. One woman telephoned recently and said, 'Could I possibly have a copy of the journals by the weekend? My husband has said at last that he will read them!' Another woman said, 'My husband is much kinder now that he knows men suffer this way as well as women!'

A teacher, an intelligent woman, would not remain in a shop unless she clasped in her hand a toy car to remind her of her own car parked nearby, should she feel forced to leave in a hurry. When I mention this woman, listeners are often amused. It is because of such anticipated ridicule that sufferers from agoraphobia are reluctant to confess their fears even to their families or friends. And though a husband may begin by sympathizing with his wife, he may eventually become irritated, critical, and finally desperate at the inconveniences the illness brings. And yet the wife will struggle on heroically, understanding these difficulties only too well, and feeling desperately guilty because of them.

PLANS ARE MADE, BROKEN; REMADE, REBROKEN

Contemplating taking an agoraphobic wife on holiday is especially frustrating and exhausting. One minute she says she will go; the next that she cannot make it. So plans are made, broken; remade, rebroken. Bookings are made and cancelled several times, with many a deposit forfeited in the meantime. No small part of a husband's frustration lies in his swinging from optimism at some apparent improvement in his wife's condition to despair when she slips into setback, and usually for no reason that makes sense to him.

The wife also has her share of frustration, especially if, because of his disappointment or lack of interest, her husband fails to give the co-operation she craves. She feels this acutely because frustration, like so many of her emotions, is exaggerated by sensitization. She may think he is wittingly unco-operative, and in a moment of despair thinks she hates him. Indeed, she is sometimes bewildered by the depth of her antipathy and resentment. Although she knows the old love must be there, she cannot *feel* it. She thinks in confusion, 'What is reality, my present dislike, or my old love?' She is especially frightened because she feels the dislike so convincingly. One wife wrote, 'It is as if I am just about to see through a mist of unreality, but never quite make it. I don't know if I really love my husband, because I see him now as another person, not the man I married.'

'ROLL OVER AND GO TO SLEEP!'

Another woman said, 'D., who used to be such a marvellous help, has reached the stage of "do it yourself" and I don't get much help from him now. If I have a turn during the night, his pat solution to the whole thing is, "Roll over and go to sleep!" Doesn't he know by now, if I could roll over and sleep, I would?'

'IF THEY ONLY KNEW!'

Here again, understanding that inability to feel love is a usual but temporary result of emotional exhaustion helps cheer the sufferer and ease bewilderment and guilt. One should not sigh too deeply for a family's understanding, nor pity oneself and think, 'If only they knew!' Very few families 'know' and most sufferers follow the same lonely road hedged by misunderstanding. Waste no strength on self-pity. It is an expensive emotion; it robs you of the will to go forward and never cured anyone.

Also, do not be too upset if you are told you could recover if you really wanted to. Be consoled: I have rarely met the nervously ill man or woman who had no wish to recover. He or she may have failed so often in the attempt that the will to get better seems dead. However, it usually smoulders on, ready to rise again for another valiant, if misdirected, effort. Let there be no misunderstanding about this: the vast majority of my nervously ill patients (and I do not use the word 'vast' lightly) yearn to recover. Of course there is the occasional work-dodger who prefers to retreat into illness rather than face the responsibilities of ordinary living. In my practice such cases have been rare.

'AM I TO ESCAPE SOMETHING, DOCTOR?'

Some people ask anxiously, 'Am I really trying to escape from something, Doctor? My last doctor said this, but what am I trying to escape from?' This inquiry often comes from women who want desperately to be shown how to recover. If the husband believes his wife is trying to escape into illness to gain his attention, her desperation is pitiable. Any sensible person would want to escape from, not into, agoraphobia – or any anxiety state – and the majority of my nervously ill patients have been sensible. They have proved this by the lives they have led after recovery.

During the last two years, I have written a quarterly journal for 1,300 sufferers from an anxiety state in many different countries. The majority have agoraphobia as part of their illness. Had I not been convinced they wanted to, and could, be cured – even by the remote control of journals alone (I have not met these people) – I would not have spent so much time and effort writing and distributing the journals. Many of these men and women have recently sent in most satisfyingly successful reports of their progress. The eight journals are included in this book.

If you are reading this to find help for your nerves, but can move freely – do not suffer from agoraphobia – do not be disappointed because I have talked so much about fear of leaving the safety of home. In the following chapters you will find many of your fears, symptoms and experiences explained, and treatment advised.

If agoraphobia is part of your illness, be assured, it can be cured. And now, how to cure it and other nervous suffering.

✤

CHAPTER 3

Cure of Physical Nervous
Symptoms binding Housewife
to House, Executive to City

If some problem, guilt, sorrow or disgrace, has caused illness and is now helping to keep you sensitized, naturally this must be coped with before you can fully recover.

However, even here, understanding your physical symptoms and knowing how to cope with them – as advised in the following chapters – will help you find some peace and so enable you to give more attention to your problem. In addition, solving the apparently insoluble problem is discussed in Chapter 5.

Each sufferer, whether with or without a special problem keeping him ill, should learn how to:

✤ Cope with his nervous symptoms – panic, palpitations, weakness, and so on.

✤ Cope with any upsetting nervous experiences accompanying his illness – such as loss of confidence, feelings of unreality, obsession, depression.

You may think, 'That's a lot to do before I can be cured!' However exacting the programme may seem to you, cure depends on four simple rules:

1. Face, do not run away.
2. Accept, do not fight.
3. Float past, do not arrest and listen-in.
4. Let time pass, do not be impatient with time.

In my earlier book *Self Help for Your Nerves* I wrote: 'When you see these four rules, you may think, "This is too simple for me!" Despite what you think now, you may need to study these rules carefully before you will know how to apply them successfully. Indeed, it is enlightening to see how many people sink deeper and deeper into their illness by doing the exact opposite.

'The nervously ill person usually notices each new symptom in alarm, listens-in in apprehension, and yet at the same time is afraid to examine it too closely for fear he will make it worse. He agitatedly seeks occupation to try to force forgetfulness. *This is running away, not facing.*

'He may try to cope with the unwelcome feelings by tensing himself against them, thinking, "I must not let this get the better of me!" *He is fighting, not accepting and floating.*

'Also he keeps looking back and worrying because so much time has passed and he is not yet cured, as if there were an evil spirit which could be exorcised if only he, or the doctor, knew how to do it. *He is impatient with time; not willing to let time pass.*

'Need we be impressed if he thinks it will take something more drastic than facing, accepting, floating and letting time pass to cure him? I don't think we need.'

The symptoms discussed here are those that most often deter the nervously ill person from venturing out alone: panic (above all); attacks of palpitation; fairly constant quickly beating heart; 'missed' heartbeats; giddiness; weak turns; a feeling of inability to take in a deep breath – and this includes a fear of suffocation; fear of vomiting in front of others; feeling of 'a lump in the throat' usually accompanied by difficulty in swallowing solid food (especially embarrassing when dining out); trembling hands; deep blushing. A sufferer may have only a few of these symptoms, very few have all of them.

The most common experiences are: indecision; suggestibility; loss of confidence; feelings of unreality, of personality disintegration; that dreaded early morning feeling; strange thoughts; obsession; depression.

These symptoms and experiences may be found in any anxiety state, of which fear of leaving the safety of home may, or may not, be a part. So if you are nervously ill but can move freely from home, you will still find most of your distressing physical nervous symptoms explained and treated here.

PANIC

Understanding the anxiety state based primarily on fear of the symptoms of fear (the kind I am discussing here) depends fundamentally on understanding panic, because without the recurring lash of panic nerves would calm and other nervous symptoms would then be less intense.

Panic is particularly dominating in agoraphobia and to avoid panicking while out, an agoraphobic woman may arrange special props. Some push a perambulator, others lead a dog on a leash, some wear dark glasses. Many prefer to go out at night, or in the rain, because they feel less conspicuous and expect to meet fewer people. Such subterfuge gives a certain protection and support, and in this way the sufferer may eventually gain enough courage to venture further and further from home. However, the woman who recovers like this does not fully understand how she is recovering, so there may be that constant menacing thought, 'What if it were to come back?' Since *it* is fear – stress – itself, as long as she is afraid of *it* returning, *it* is already on its way; even while out, she is keeping the home fires burning.

Props Have a Habit of Giving Way

Also, props have a habit of giving way. The surest way to permanent recovery is to know how to face, and truly accept, fear and not placate it with subterfuge. How simple this sounds; how difficult it can be, and how much support and encouragement the sufferer rightly feels he or she needs while carrying out this apparently simple task.

At the Mercy of 'Some Thing'

One of the keys to understanding sensitization lies in realizing that, in a sensitized person, simply thinking of panic may bring it, or that panic may seem to come unbidden. This is why the sufferer often feels caught in a trap. He will say, 'The panic comes so quickly, I can't do anything about it.' Hence his constant watchfulness to leave a way open for quick retreat and his finding eventually that going out alone, or leaving the home town, with the threat of panic 'round the corner', may become too frightening to be contemplated.

It helps to understand such fear if I compare our automatic nerves with the trigger of a gun. A rusty trigger is stiff to pull; when well oiled, well used, it responds more readily to the touch. The 'nerve-trigger' of the woman wearing dark glasses and valiantly pushing a perambulator before her is so well used it fires off (and 'fire' is a good word) at even the mere sight of a neighbour to whom she may have to stop and speak. This is especially upsetting, because *she used not to feel this way*. Of course not; when she was not sensitized, an inquisitive neighbour's approach meant, at most, only annoyance, never this flashing fear.

Reducing Panic to Normal Intensity

Cure lies in developing such insulation to panic that it comes neither so readily nor so acutely. In other words, cure lies in reducing panic to normal intensity and frequency. To do this, the nervous person must understand that when he panics, he feels not one fear, as he supposes, but two separate fears. I call these the *first* and *second* fear.

The importance of recognizing these two separate fears cannot be overestimated because although the sensitized person may have no control over the *first* fear, with understanding and practice he can learn how to control the *second* fear, and it is this *second* fear that is keeping the first alive, keeping him sensitized, nervously ill.

First Fear

Each of us experiences *first* fear from time to time. It is the fear that comes almost reflexly in response to danger. It is normal in intensity; we understand it and accept it because we know that when the danger passes, the fear will also pass. The flash of *first* fear that comes to a sensitized person in response to danger can be so electric in its swiftness, so out of proportion to the danger causing it, that he cannot readily dismiss it. Indeed, he usually recoils from it, and as he recoils he adds a second flash of fear. *He adds fear of the first fear.* Indeed, he may be much more concerned with the physical feeling of panic than with the original danger. And because that old bogey, sensitization, prolongs the first flash, the second flash may seem to join it. This is why the two fears feel as one.

A flash of *first* fear can come in response to a thought only vaguely understood; to some mildly unpleasant memory; or, as mentioned earlier, it may seem to come unbidden. Can you see how easily victimized a sensitized person can be by *first* fear?

All the symptoms of stress – the pounding heart, churning stomach, trembling body and so on – can be called *first* fear, because they too seem to come unbidden, like the flash of panic that comes in response to danger, and to these symptoms the nervously ill person certainly adds much *second* fear.

Second Fear

Pages could be filled with examples of *second* fear and I doubt if there would be one that some of you have not known at some time. Recognizing *second* fear is easier when we realize it can be prefixed by 'Oh, my goodness!' and 'What if ... ?' 'Oh, my goodness, it took three capsules to get me to sleep last night! What if three don't work tonight?' 'What if I get worse, not better?' So many Oh, my goodnesses, so many What ifs, make up *second* fear. You probably know them all.

Nervously ill people, hemmed in at the school meeting, church, in the cinema, in a restaurant, have only to feel trapped to flash *first* fear – to which they immediately add *second* fear, as they think, 'Oh, my goodness, here it is again! I can't stand it. I'll make a fool of myself in front of all these people! Let me out of here! Quickly! Quickly! Quickly!' With each 'quickly' they become more and more tense, and as the tension mounts, naturally the panic mounts, until they wonder how much longer they can hold on without cracking. So, they take an even tighter grip on themselves and build up even more tension as the moments pass. Mounting tension is alarming and exhausting. It is difficult to hold tensely on to oneself for a few minutes, and yet, at the school meeting, in church, these people try to hold tensely on to themselves for an hour or more. Small wonder the panic grows, until they are terrified of what crisis it may bring. They are sure there must be a crisis in which 'something terrible' will happen and vaguely see themselves 'collapsing'. They are never sure what this 'something terrible' might be, but feel it hovering menacingly in the background. They can be reassured. There is a limit to the intensity in a spasm of panic even a sensitized body can produce and they have probably experienced it already. However, they do not realize this because their imagination is working overtime.

The Mind Goes Numb

Their fear is so acute, and their imagination so active, that at the peak of panic they feel the mind goes numb, feel they can neither think nor act clearly. This is why keeping a way open for quick retreat — sitting near the exit — seems so imperative. These nervously ill people do not understand that it is the fears they add themselves, the succession of *second* fears, that may finally drive them to find refuge outside the building.

And when outside, they will probably feel relieved, breathe freely for a while. But as soon as they face the fact that they failed once more, they despair, because they think they will never, never, be able to sit through another such function. They gave themselves an impossible task; they went through every moment heroically, *but they did it the wrong way*.

If you sometimes seek refuge outside a hall, ask yourself why you can gradually relax when outside, yet cannot do so while inside. You will say, 'As soon as I am outside, I feel different.' The truth is, as soon as you are outside, you think differently, so of course you feel better.

He Always Manages to Say, 'Excuse Me, Please!'

When you are sensitized, feeling follows thought so swiftly and intensely that you may be afraid, while sitting at the school function, of what you may think, and afraid of what you may then feel. But you do think, don't you? A very vivid imagination is well at work and sometimes you can almost see yourself becoming hysterical and being led outside. Yet I have never seen or heard of a nervously ill person becoming hysterical at a function. When he or she decides he cannot stand another minute and leaves the hall, he always manages to say, 'Excuse me, please!' to the person beside him.

Exactly what does happen outside the building that makes outside so much more bearable than inside? If you are the person in this situation you probably think 'Thank goodness, nothing can happen now!' and you release that tense hold on yourself. First, you let it go in thought, and this eases the tense, physical hold. If you could do the same inside the hall, your problem would be solved. It would, you know. It may seem more complicated than this to you, but it isn't. And yet, what sounds so simple to say is not so simple to do.

First Fear Must Always Die Down

How are you to cope with that feeling of panic, those frightening thoughts, that agitation, inside the hall? You cope by practising seeing panic through, even seeing agitation through, with as much acceptance as you can muster. It is all those Oh, my goodnesses, all those What ifs, that build up into what you call a turn, a crisis. Try to understand that your body is not a machine; that it has a limited capacity to produce adrenalin; that therefore *first* fear can come only in a wave and must always die down *if you but wait* and do not fall into the trap of stoking your fires with more and more *second* fear and so, more and more adrenalin. If you remain seated and relax to the best of your ability – even allow your body to slump in the chair – and are prepared to let the panic flash, let it do its very worst without withdrawing tensely from it, *there will be no mounting panic*. Your sensitized body may continue to flash fear from time to time, *but the panic will not mount*, and at least you will be able to see the function through.

Must you let these physical feelings hold such terror? Must you let them, horrible though they may be, spoil your life while the way to calm them is within your own power? Think about this and understand that *you are bluffed by physical feelings* of no great medical significance. This realization alone has cured some people.

If you are prepared to practise seeing panic through, this acceptance, shaky as it may be at first, will bring some peace, enough to lessen the flow of adrenalin and so begin desensitization. It is bombardment by *second* fear, day after day, month after month, for one reason or another, that keeps nerves alerted, always triggered to fire that *first* fear so intensely.

A Small Voice Says, 'Go On!'

Your willingness to try to see panic through means that at least some part of you is going forward. A small voice says, 'Go on!' despite a stronger, more persistent voice saying, 'No, I can't.' You build on that little voice. However faint it may be, it is the seed of acceptance, the beginning of cure.

Even when you succeed in coping with *second* fear, desensitization takes time. With utter acceptance, a sensitized body may still flash *first* fear for some time to come. Some patients have complained that although they no longer panic, they have an inner feeling of apprehension, almost of vibration, as if panic were on the verge of coming. This can be compared to the vibrations of a large bell after it has been struck and the sound dies away.

Although disturbing, one can learn to function with this feeling of inner vibration, near-panic. It gradually passes.

A woman wrote, 'I soon learned to disregard the trembling feeling that came after the panic ceased. It did not last long.' Sensitized nerves heal as naturally as a broken leg; but it takes time. To face and accept one's nervous symptoms without adding *second* fear – how important this is. It works miracles, if one is prepared to do just this.

It is not easy to face, accept and let time pass. It is especially difficult to let time pass, because so much time has already been spent in suffering and despair that asking for more time to pass may seem an impossible demand. It is difficult but necessary.

Also, don't think I underestimate the severity of your panic. I understand how severe it can be and I also know that even with the help of daily sedation and the best of intentions and determination to accept, you may think yourself too exhausted to do so. It is as if your mind is willing to accept, but your body is too tired to take its orders.

You may, while recovering, have the strange experience of feeling panic and other nervous symptoms, and yet, at the same time, know *they no longer matter*. One sufferer wrote, 'I still suffered from agoraphobia, but I was not afraid of that any more. It was just a nuisance.' In other words, the feelings lingered because of memory and some remaining sensitization, but she knew how to deal with them.

However long you have been ill, if you make up your mind not to add *second* fear, complete recovery is inevitable. How important it is to unmask panic and see those two separate fears. How important to learn how to recognize *second* fear and send it packing. Recognizing *second* fear and coping with it is the way to desensitization, the way to recovery. I assure you of this.

'Putting Up With'

You must be sure you know the difference between true acceptance and just 'putting up with'. 'Putting up with' means withdrawing from panic in panic; adding panic to panic; hoping that panic will go quickly and not come back – sometimes even hoping it will come so that you can get it over. It means avoiding people and places that bring panic, so that the horizon becomes narrower and narrower, until it is eventually bounded by the front gate. It means always leaving a way open for quick retreat; it means expecting retreat; it means continued illness.

Acceptance

True acceptance means recognizing *second* fear and adding as little of it as possible. Recognizing *second* fear may not be easy at first, but when you are familiar with it, you will be amazed how much *second* fear you have been adding as torture to your daily life. True acceptance means even welcoming panic so you can practise coping with it the way I have advised, until it no longer frightens. I can almost hear your groans as you read this, but *you can do it*. I have watched too many people, just as desperate as you and with no more courage than you think you have, come through panic to peace; so why shouldn't you?

'This Doctor Doesn't Know How Sick I Am!'

Do not be tempted to think, 'This doctor doesn't know how sick I am!' Can you see how, by thinking this way, you have already added *second* fear? How insidious that *second* fear can be! When you finally learn to see panic through with true acceptance, you do not need dark glasses; do not have to sit at the back of the hall; do not have to walk as far as the corner of the street one week, into the village the next, before you finally graduate to the supermarket. You could go by bus to the town centre today, because by learning how to cope with panic, you take your cure with you wherever you go.

So:

❧ Remember, props have a habit of giving way, so do not placate fear with excuses – face and truly accept it.

❧ Learn to recognize *second* fear and practise sending it packing.

❧ Wait. Do not stoke your fire with *second* fear by tensely withdrawing from panic.

❧ There is a limit to the intensity of panic even a sensitized body can produce.

❧ Your mind does not go numb. You can always think, if only the wrong thoughts.

- You have been bluffed by physical feelings. *First* fear will always die down if you give it time.
- Let *first* fear do its worst and there will be no mounting panic.

Build on that little voice.

PALPITATIONS

By palpitations, I mean the short abrupt attack of rapidly beating heart that may come occasionally to a nervously ill person. It may occur on exertion, or perhaps just as he is dropping off to, or awakening from, sleep.

Palpitations, when one is in bed and alone at night, can be especially alarming. All too often, the victim immediately sits up in a panic or lies sweating, hands tingling, face burning, while he waits for some further development which, he suspects, could even be death. The anxiety of weeks, months, may have so sensitized his heart that any noise, any stress – perhaps merely the slamming of a car door in the street or an uneasy dream, anything which wakens him with a start – may be enough to set his heart racing.

If you suffer in this way and are awakened by palpitations, the more you panic, the more adrenalin is released and the longer the attack can last. Although you may think, 'I wish Doctor could feel my pulse now, this is terrifying!' were you to take your pulse, you would find your heart is not beating at much more than a hundred and twenty beats each minute. If any one of us runs for a bus when out of form, our heart may beat just as quickly as during palpitations and we may be just as conscious of its pounding; but it does not worry us because we understand the cause and know the rapid beating will ease when we stop running.

Most people are frightened by a sudden attack of palpitations, but nervous palpitations are not at all dangerous. The full, bursting feeling in the throat is only the unusually strong pulsation of the main arteries in the neck. If you could see how thick, and appreciate how powerful your heart muscle is, you would lose all fear of its bursting or being damaged by palpitations. A healthy heart can tolerate a rate of over two hundred beats per minute for days, even weeks, without any damage. So let your heart race until it chooses to calm down, remembering that it is a good heart, beating quickly because of nervous stimulation; that such stimulation will not harm it, and that it will always eventually calm down. I am assuming that your doctor has examined your heart and told you your trouble is 'only nerves', that 'there is nothing wrong with your heart'.

Understanding that palpitations are no more than a temporary upset in the timing of the heartbeats caused by overstimulated nerves, and that the attack always calms down, will help you lose your fear of them. Less fear means less adrenalin and consequently less excitation, so the attacks come less frequently, and, as your health improves, finally cease to come. At all costs resist treating yourself as an invalid.

If you have an attack while out, you may feel more comfortable if you rest until the attack passes. However, you may continue walking or working, if you prefer to do so. While you wait, or walk, try to accept the palpitations without recoiling from them, remembering that even while your heart palpitates nature is working to calm its racing. So, *do not turn homewards in fear*. There is no need to hurry home to rest after an attack. I stress once more that I give this advice only to those whose doctor has examined the heart, and told them their trouble is nervous.

If you are agoraphobic, never let fear of palpitations send you hurrying home. Stay in the shop; at the school meeting; in the cinema. Nature will stop the attack in her own time; *you* do not have to do anything about it, except willingly see it through. If you do this, you will be surprised how soon the nervous palpitations will pass.

During recovery, some people learn to accept their palpitations so well they can turn over and go to sleep during an attack. Others need a pill to help calm them, and I sometimes advise this during the early stages of recovery. I do not ask for stoical forbearance from a severely sensitized person. In the beginning, I ask only for an understanding of the harmless nature of nervous palpitations, and as much acceptance with as little panic as possible.

CONSTANTLY QUICKLY BEATING HEART

A person under the tension of sustained anxiety may find his heart constantly beating quickly, although not as fast as during an attack of palpitations. As with palpitations, the increased rate is merely nervous reaction and once again it is the awareness that disturbs, not the actual rate. This constant awareness of the body repeatedly brings the sick person's thoughts back to himself and he dreads this. His thoughts so often, and too easily, revert to himself. With the most courageous intentions, the woman afraid to leave the house alone may venture out thinking, 'I'll really try to make the corner shop today and I'm not going to think about myself!' So, as she walks, she concentrates with great effort on her neighbours' gardens, passing cars, and once inside the shop, while waiting to be served, glues her eyes to the tins on the shelves and reads each label as it has never been read before. And yet all the time she feels her heart beating quickly, her body trembling, her legs shaking, until she wonders how much longer she can bear it. The body works on the mind, and the mind then works on the body: the old cycle of despair that may finally drive her out of the shop unserved.

Afraid to Notice What is Happening to Her Body

She has been resorting to subterfuge to take her mind off her feelings. That is running away, not facing. No one can work the miracle of calming the body while he is afraid to notice what is happening to it. While her body is sensitized this woman will feel her heart beating quickly and she will remain sensitized to the beating while she anxiously listens to, and records, each beat, or just as anxiously tries not to listen

No Magic Switch to Calm Your Heart Immediately

If you suffer in this way, be prepared to live with this quick beating, to accept the racing, thumping, as part of the process of recovery, until your nerves become less sensitized. You have made the mistake of thinking that while your heart continues to beat quickly, you must still be ill. It may be weeks before you cease to be conscious of your heart's quick action, but once you accept it, *you will be getting better all the time.* There is no magic switch to calm your heart immediately, although sedatives help.*

---

* Drugs called beta-blockers are used today (1987) to slow the rate of a 'nervous' heart. The smallest effective dose should be used for a short time. Consult your doctor.

A constantly quick pulse may have a physical cause; for example, anaemia, or an overactive thyroid gland. So once again be sure you have your doctor's assurance that your quick rate is nervous.

'MISSED' HEARTBEATS

A heart stimulated by too much alcohol, nicotine, caffeine (coffee, tea), irritated by indigestion, or simply under nervous tension, may 'miss' beats. The beats are not really missed, although they feel like this. They are spaced irregularly and are called extrasystoles. Once again, the timing of the beat is at fault. The heart compensates for an unusually quick beat by taking a restful pause, so that the three unevenly spaced beats take the same time as three even beats. The long pause gives the sensation of the heart 'stopping' or 'missing' a beat. It doesn't.

'Missed' beats are not dangerous. Most people over forty, and many healthy young people, have them but are unaware of them. In the sensitized person, the forceful beat after the long pause may bring an unpleasant feeling – rather like a sudden descent in a lift – and this can be very disconcerting if there is a long run of extrasystoles, and especially if attacks occur frequently. The sufferer may stand still, thinking his heart is about to stop. The heart will not stop because of 'missed' beats.

Indigestion – wind around the heart – can aggravate this condition. Exercise abolishes nervous extrasystoles, so do not let them intimidate you into lying on the couch.

Some sufferers describe their 'missed' beats as fibrillation. Fibrillation is quite different from extrasystoles. Get your doctor's reassurance about this, if you have any doubt.

GIDDINESS

When a housebound person is trying to go out alone, there is nothing more discouraging than a footpath that seems to heave, houses that sway, and a body that feels unsteady. The usual response is to sit down and wait for the giddiness to pass, or if no seat is available, to hold on to the nearest support and later to return home and give up trying to leave the house that day. Indeed, giddiness may be such a frequent visitor to the nervously ill woman even at home, that waiting for a day when she can go out not feeling giddy may mean being housebound for weeks. Hence the plaintive question, 'How can I ever leave the house while I am as giddy as this? I have only to think of going out and I am worse.'

There are two kinds of giddiness. One, called vertigo, is usually not 'nervous' in origin. With true vertigo stationary objects seem to move rapidly, the room to swirl suddenly. The sufferer may stagger so violently he may be thrown to the floor. There is usually an organic cause for such violent giddiness – perhaps a small piece of wax stuck to the eardrum, a blocked eustachian tube, and so on. The sufferer eventually consults a doctor.

We are rarely concerned with true vertigo in nervous illness. Here, giddiness is more likely to be the lightheaded type. The sufferer feels 'floaty', giddy within himself, and is not so conscious of everything spinning violently around. Nervous giddiness is tension giddiness. Tension interferes with the balancing mechanism (semi-circular canals) receiving the correct messages from eye, neck and body muscles. Although the interference may sometimes be so severe that the victim may feel propelled by it, the feeling of propulsion is never as acute as with true vertigo.

The swaying type of giddiness may also accompany low blood pressure, or may be felt when high blood pressure temporarily falls; for example, in hot weather, after taking sleeping pills, and so on. It is reassuring to know that giddiness more often follows a fall, than a rise, in blood pressure. So many people with high blood pressure, when they have a spell of giddiness, are unnecessarily afraid of a stroke.

'Change of life' may also bring giddy spells; as may bending while gardening, typing, or washing hair, or simply rising too quickly from the horizontal position. Most mechanisms misbehave sometimes, so why should we expect a machine as complicated as our body to always function perfectly? As it is, the body gradually adjusts itself to tension giddiness, and it will do so more quickly if we do not add further tension by being afraid of the giddiness. One woman was haunted by the thought of being held up in her car by the red light at intersections. As soon as the green changed to amber she would think, 'I daren't stop now! This is where I always have a giddy spell!' So she would rush through the crossing on the amber light, and of course, this extra tension accentuated any tendency to giddiness. *She had induced her own giddiness.*

Another woman said she was too giddy to walk up the road, but she could manage very well on her bicycle. She had been able to convince herself she was not giddy while riding because she did not have as much opportunity to concentrate on herself while riding as she did when walking, and consequently was not as giddy. Attitude of mind can work wonders.

INABILITY TO TAKE A DEEP BREATH

So many over-anxious people, especially when out, find expanding their chest to take in a deep breath disturbingly difficult. This does not mean their lungs or heart are diseased, merely that chest muscles are overtensed. They do not understand this feeling and 'gasp and gulp' for breath – as one woman described it – half believing that unless they succeed, they will suffocate.

Nature was not so foolish as to put on to our conscious effort the full responsibility of breathing; if she had, how would we breathe while asleep, or when unconscious? We have a respiratory centre in our brain which automatically regulates our breathing. If we do not inspire enough oxygen, carbon dioxide accumulates in our blood and when it reaches a certain concentration this stimulates the breathing centre which then, by means of our involuntary nerves, forcibly expands our lungs to take in more air and wash out the excess carbon dioxide.

To illustrate how automatically this centre works, I ask a patient, disturbed in this way, to see how long he can hold his breath; to actually stop breathing. At first he may be reluctant to try such a 'dangerous' experiment, but when he does, he is surprised to find that after about half a minute – the time for carbon dioxide to accumulate – he is forced to breathe almost against his will, and then by taking a very deep breath indeed. When he realizes there is a control beyond his control, he usually sees the folly of his desperate struggle.

If you suffer with nervous 'overbreathing' do not let it frighten you. Breathe as shallowly as you feel you must, but do not be concerned with what will happen because you breathe this way. Your respiratory centre will see that you inspire enough air, despite your effort to hinder it.

Let this automatic control look after you. It guards you very well at night while you sleep, so why should it fail during the day? It will not fail.

Shallow breathing can temporarily wash out too much carbon dioxide and so the sufferer may feel giddy, his hands may tingle. This is not a threat of a stroke. It means only that the blood has become slightly alkaline because of reduced carbon dioxide, and the body responds to increased alkalinity with giddiness and tingling. The respiratory centre gradually adjusts this by slowing down breathing until enough carbon dioxide has accumulated to correct the excess alkalinity.

I have sometimes been surprised at how quickly a patient can recover from shallow breathing when he loses his fear of it. A young woman walked into my consulting room, breathing in obvious distress. She was desperate because, as she said, she had been breathing this way on and off for months. My explanation of the respiratory centre, and then the experiment of holding her breath, relieved her mind so much that she relaxed and began to take deep natural breaths. She has not been troubled by shallow breathing since then.

Do not be disappointed if, despite understanding, you still have occasional difficulty in breathing deeply. It is not important. Acceptance (real acceptance) once more works the miracle by releasing tension.*

---

* A good exercise to stop rapid shallow breathing (hyperventilation): lie flat on floor or bed, bend knees and bring legs close to your body, keeping feet flat on ground. Then place arms across chest, right hand grasping left shoulder, left hand grasping right shoulder. This produces abdominal breathing.

WEAKNESS ('JELLY-LEGS')

The weakness that comes with nervous disturbance is the weakness of emotional shock – the weakness that any one of us might feel if told suddenly we had inherited a million. Adrenalin, released by shock, dilates blood vessels in leg muscles, so that blood drains from the rest of our body into these muscles and does not circulate adequately. This brings a feeling of trembling weakness in our legs. After an asthmatic patient has had an injection of adrenalin, he, or she, may have to rest until the trembling and the weakness – the after-effects of adrenalin – pass.

The agoraphobic woman may have little spasms of panic whenever she thinks of going out alone; so, when she starts off, she is already in such a state that any extra strain while out – crossing a main road, standing in a queue, entering a bus – may immediately bring a feeling of trembling weakness: her legs seem to turn to jelly, ready to buckle under her. So she thinks, 'What is the use of trying today? I might as well go home.'

It is not difficult to understand why, if she does venture out again, she will begin by timidly testing herself to see if she can get as far as the front gate, then to the end of the street and so on, without feeling weak. The fear she feels while trying in this way is an open invitation to the feelings she dreads. She has placed herself in the cycle of fear-adrenalin-fear. Just as realization that they have been bluffed by physical feelings has cured some patients, so has understanding of the fear-adrenalin-fear cycle.

The nervously ill person sitting in a hall surrounded by people continuously gives himself little shocks (extra adrenalin) by thinking, 'How much longer can I go through this! What if I faint! I can feel it coming!' – shock after shock. He can usually take onslaught upon onslaught, at worst feeling light-headed. The nervously ill person rarely faints. So relax in this knowledge if in a situation where you feel 'weak all over'.

A Pilgrimage from Chair to Chair

A nervous woman may tire so easily that standing while shopping, especially waiting to be served, is an ordeal. Shopping becomes a pilgrimage from chair to chair. If no chair is handy, her immediate apprehension of a weak turn is enough to invite one.

If the shopper is prepared to stand, or walk, without apprehension, however 'charged with lead' her legs may feel she will find by the time she has finished that not only will she have recovered, but she will have gained confidence from the effort. As long as she stays apprehensive fear continues to release adrenalin and the weakness persists. By disregarding weakness, she will find that strength gradually returns.

If you suffer from recurring attacks of nervous weakness, try to remember the less you worry about your wobbly legs, the less wobbly they will be. Jelly-legs will still carry you, if you let them; so give them the chance. If your legs feel weak, it is because they are responding normally to the tension you have been building up. The weakness and heaviness are only feelings. This is not true organic weakness. So once more do not be bluffed by physical feelings.

She Sent Her Legs the Wrong Messages

The importance of attitude is well illustrated by one woman who can walk confidently on grass, but feels her legs 'give way' when she walks on hard pavement. On grass she, perhaps subconsciously, sends her legs the message, 'You can walk here', and of course, they can. On pavement, she sends them the signal, 'You can't walk here', and her legs react accordingly.

Possibly she has had her first attack of weakness while walking on a pavement and memory, even subconsciously, may linger to rob her of confidence when walking on a hard surface; or the jarring impact of her heels against the pavement may make her conscious of her legs, and so of her fear. This may sound childish, but when a woman (or man) has been through as many weak turns over the years as this woman, the old tracks of suffering respond uncomfortably readily and despair follows just as easily. It takes special courage and understanding to come out of such an emotional quagmire. But if you suffer this way, you can do it. A change in attitude, even though tentative at first, gradually brings a change in strength. Our nervous control of muscles is a double-edged weapon. Muscles strengthen to the right attitude, tremble to the wrong.

We Keep Our Grip by Letting it Go

It is strange how we keep a grip on ourselves *by being prepared to release it*. We cannot keep the right kind of grip by tensely holding on, as so many wrongly suppose. By abandoning ourselves to whatever our body may care to do, we release the tension that fatigues the nerves controlling muscles and blood-vessels, so that they recover their ability to function normally, and strength gradually returns. *So much of a nervously ill person's suffering is self- induced through ignorance*. It is also induced by the hovering shadow of having to some day, somehow, face what they feel is the *ultimate*. No one is quite sure what he means by this, but each is convinced it is crucial. The *ultimate* – in other words, the worst that could possibly happen – is no more than fear and imagination working together to create a bogeyman which will disappear if one has the courage to confront it.

While a sufferer reading this at home may feel hopeful and be prepared to face the worst, it is not so easy to stay reassured during an attack of weakness away from home. The despair of the moment may be so acute, it is difficult to reassure oneself adequately during that moment. If only one's body would respond quickly to one's own reassurance! Instead, it may take quite a while to recover from an attack of weakness. Also, even with understanding and acceptance, because of previous months of tension, weak spells may recur from time to time. This is also part of the strangeness of recovery.

It is only human to remain a little afraid of weak turns and so unwittingly pave the way for their recurrence. Do not be deterred by nervous weakness. Muscles and attitude of mind both strengthen with use.

Some people faint more easily than others, whether nervously ill or not; for example, soldiers are known to faint on parade when they must stand still for long periods, especially in hot weather. This kind of faintness can be corrected by moving one's body as much as the situation permits, and so keeping blood circulating. Please do not think, after reading this, that if you have to stand still for any length of time you must immediately begin to fidget. The nervously ill person who stands quite still for longer than a few moments would be hard to find.

TOO LITTLE SUGAR IN THE BLOOD

Occasionally a nervously ill, or indeed a non-nervously ill person uses up the body's available glucose too rapidly and the level of blood sugar falls below normal. Weakness with trembling and sweating may then follow. The nervous person may blame his nerves for this. While these attacks do come from working strenuously, under pressure, especially if one has not had enough to eat during the day, they are not necessarily part of nervous illness, and are relieved by eating something sweet. If no food is available, simply resting for ten minutes gives the liver time to release stored glycogen, which is then broken down into glucose. If these turns come frequently, the sufferer should plan his diet to include enough protein – meat, fish, cheese, eggs. The attacks are called hypoglycaemia.

So:

- ✗ Do not be drawn to every chair you see, however charged with lead your legs may feel.
- ✗ Remember, apprehension releases the adrenalin that helps to bring weakness.
- ✗ Jelly-legs will still carry you, if you will let them.
- ✗ You keep the best grip by being prepared to release it.

FEAR OF VOMITING

I have not known one nervously ill person who has vomited in public. However, some are so haunted by this fear they refuse invitations to eat with friends or attend any public gathering. Many have gagged gently to themselves, or hurriedly left the room to do so outside, but vomit – no. This is surely consoling when we realize that short of putting his finger down his throat, a nervous person could hardly stimulate his vomiting muscles more than he does by his anxious concentration on them. It is not as easy as a nervous person imagines for a healthy stomach, even a nervous stomach, to regurgitate its food. As I mentioned earlier, it is the tense holding on that does the damage, not the letting go. If the nervous person were to give up the struggle to prevent vomiting, his stomach muscles would gradually relax and not only would he lose his squeamish feeling but vomiting would be even less likely.

Feel as nauseated and as sick as you must while in the company of others, but be reassured, if you accept this you will not vomit.

DIFFICULTY IN SWALLOWING

The 'lump in the throat' mentioned earlier may be most troublesome at mealtimes. The sufferer is sure he cannot swallow solid food, or at least finds this difficult.

I keep biscuits in my office especially for such a patient. Biscuits are dry, and at the sight of one the patient usually recoils. When I ask him to chew one, he says, 'I couldn't swallow a biscuit. I'd never get it down!' I remind him that I asked him to chew, not swallow. Reluctantly he bites and chews. After a while I say, 'Now remember, I want you only to chew. Don't swallow.' But already he has swallowed some of it. As soon as the moistened, softened biscuit reaches the back of the tongue, his swallowing reflexes take over and at least some of the biscuit is on its way.

You need not worry about trying to swallow; simply keep chewing. The swallowing will look after itself as the food is carried backward. And it will eventually find its way backward in spite of your nervous resistance. If you keep chewing, the food will all eventually disappear.

BLUSHING

Intense blushing can be a great trial to many young women, and even men; indeed one middle-aged man came for help saying, 'Doctor! I blush at the slightest thing. I don't just go pink. I go a deep scarlet and right down to my neck!' He, a European migrant, would not go to his club because of severe blushing. Each Saturday night he and his wife sat in loneliness – they spoke little English – although she pathetically tried to persuade him to take her to join their friends.

One woman's life became so disrupted by blushing, she would not open the door to strangers. As her husband's business was carried on partly at home, this was not only a handicap to the business, it also made her feel so shamefully inadequate that she was beginning to lose confidence in many other ways.

Her trouble began during the last war when, as a young girl, she was evacuated to a family in the country. She was a shy child and did blush a little, but at that time she gave this no special attention, until one of the older girls in the new family persisted in staring at her during meals, trying to make her blush. She was sometimes too upset to finish her meal and, of course, blushed even more profusely.

When she returned to London two years later, intense blushing had become her response to the slightest attention. She carried that cross for twenty years and was the butt of any thoughtless person who crossed her path.

She was cured at last when I explained that a blush is caused by the nerves controlling the blood vessels in our face and neck becoming so *startled* by emotion – fear, anger, shame – that they suddenly release their grip and blood floods into the vessels. Trying not to blush (and this had been her constant aim) means tensely concentrating on one's face when one should be unaware of it, and the more attention nerves get the more easily startled they become; so, of course, the more likely they are to lose their grip and bring about a blush.

When she at last understood this, I finally persuaded her to let herself blush, whatever the situation – especially at the front door – and to try not to be so upset when she did. It was not easy to persuade her she was capable of coping with this difficulty, or that doing it this way would cure her. She thought unless she took a very firm grip the blushing would surely get worse. But when I pointed out that her way of coping in the past had reduced her almost to isolation she agreed to try it my way. I also encouraged her by showing her that it was far more important not to restrict her family's life – as she was now doing – than to care about a stranger's opinion of her which, after all, was usually only one of passing attention. She finally got her priorities right and in three months was opening the front door, sometimes hardly noticing whether she blushed or not. When she saw me at that time she said she still blushed a little, but did not worry about it because her husband said a little blushing was attractive.

If blushing is your trouble, the less you care whether you blush or not, the less likely you are to blush. The difficulty is to learn not to care. The rest follows if you can manage that.

Some of the people who came to me were bewildered by interpretations made by analysts of their deep blushing, interpretations often with a sexual or guilt basis. The young woman just discussed had been told hers was due to a subconscious sexual deviation. She was happily married with children and luckily did not take this interpretation seriously. Her cure by my explanation and her courage alone showed how wrong the analyst's suggestion had been.

Interpreting deep blushing as an expression of subconscious guilt is a temptation some therapists cannot resist – unfortunately with damaging results to people for whom such interpretation is unjustified.

ANY STRANGE NEW FEELING

Beware of adding 'Oh, my goodness' to any unexpected, disturbing nervous feeling you may experience; of thinking, 'This is a new one, Doctor didn't mention this. This must be important!' It usually is not. Accept any new such feeling that may come; accept anything your body does while you walk, while you work, while you wait. I remind you it is necessary to be examined by your doctor and assured your trouble is nervous.

Understand this: You have been frightened for so long, being afraid is so much a habit, that during the early stages of recovery you will probably continue to be frightened. No one could banish fear such as yours overnight. Accept even this. Realize that for some time yet you will often add *second* fear, plenty of it. *You will add it from habit.* In the beginning you can only practise not adding it. So, when you fail, do not despair too much. Despair, yes. Who wouldn't? But don't utterly despair. The person who eventually completely recovers has learnt to disregard failure, to disregard despair.

TAKE THOSE FIRST STEPS SLOWLY

And whether agoraphobic or not, take those first steps towards recovery – whatever they may be – at a moderate pace. Do not rush. Rushing to 'get it over quickly' only increases agitation and agitation prepares the way for panic. So go slowly, gently,

Essential Help for Your Nerves

and do not be afraid to notice how you feel; do not try forcing yourself to think of something different to keep your mind off yourself – you will lose that battle for sure. How could you not notice how you feel, not think of yourself? You have been doing just this for so long, of course you will continue to do it. So accept that you may think continuously about yourself and be prepared for this also. Be prepared to think and feel anything; go towards it; do not shrink from it; and at the same time try to be not quite so impressed by the way you feel. You have been misled by feelings for such a long time. Actually, your sensitized body is functioning normally in the circumstances you are creating for it.

In circumstances of bewilderment, fear and tension such as yours, how could your heart not race, your hands not sweat, perhaps tremble; how could you not feel strange, weak, unreal? Therefore, be prepared to feel this way in the beginning and do not expect acceptance immediately to work wonders. As I said, this may be the first time in years that you have tried to go out by yourself or face other difficulties. Isn't it natural you should feel apprehensive, strange, unreal? Aren't these feelings to be expected? Of course they are. They are not even sick reactions. *They are normal reactions in the circumstances.*

Slow Recovery May Be Good For You

If you recover quickly by following this advice, that is fine. I have often seen quick recovery. However, if your recovery is slow, do not be disappointed. *Each person must be prepared to recover at his or her own pace.* Slow recovery can be good for you. It gives opportunity to practise again and again the method I teach, until you make it part of yourself. Panic rarely vanishes by suddenly ceasing to come. Panic goes only when you take the panic out of panic; that is, by seeing it through so often *without adding second fear*, that eventually even panic no longer matters.

If agoraphobic, while you move away from home, have the courage to cut the tie between yourself and the house. Release your body by thinking forward. If in a car, a bus, move forward in thought with it. Do not hold yourself back; float forward; loosen that tense hold.

In The Front Line of Battle

Practising this way could make you feel more tired and 'nervier' than ever. This is understandable. While you avoided situations where you thought you would panic, you could go weeks without panicking, but when you are willing to put yourself into fear-producing situations you are in the front line of battle as it were, and could panic now, more than you have for a long time. It is a rare person who can cope with panic the right way on every occasion in the early stages of recovery. This is why you may be temporarily more sensitized, nervier than before and so may need extra tranquillization (prescribed by your doctor) at this time. And this is why some people, when they first practise my teaching, occasionally lose heart and think they are worse, not better.

Refresh Yourself By Making No Effort

Do not be afraid to let a day or two pass without practising; do not think you will lose all you have gained if you do not practise daily. You will never lose what you have learnt, once you start to work at recovery the right way. Refreshing yourself sometimes by making no effort for a while is wiser than flogging a tired body for fear you will lose what you learnt yesterday. *Accept these halts in recovery*. I speak more about this later.

You Did Rush Headlong to Try to Get It Over

When you fail, try to discover where you went wrong. When you review the situation, I am sure you will find you did rush headlong to try to 'get it over'; you did hurry to get back home; you did withdraw in fear; did try to sit on panic, to stop it coming; did add too much *second* fear; or you were overtired and oversensitized with so much trying, so much endeavour, that you became frightened by the renewed intensity of your fear, just when you were expecting to feel better. Maybe you listened to that little voice that is always ready to discourage you; the little voice that says, 'You can never do it. The method might be right for others, but you haven't got what it takes to succeed!' How often have I heard of this little voice and how often have I seen people, frightened by it at first, eventually recover completely. Do not be influenced by that little voice. It speaks in vain to so many.

So, when you fail, go out and practise once more, but this time practise the right way. And remember, *practise, do not test yourself.* Do not think, for example, 'I went round the park so well last week, I wonder how I'll do it today', and then be disappointed if you are more afraid today than you were last week. Your anxiety to do as well as you did last week could make you begin the journey round the park just a little more fearfully than you did a week ago, so that it takes only a minor incident to throw you into panic and to instantly bring disappointment. The way to recovery is rather tricky, isn't it? Especially if you take every baffling twist and turn seriously. Accept it all. Do not waste energy trying to work out why you managed so well one day, so badly the next. Accept it, until the meaning of true acceptance is written on your heart.

Following this advice is not easy, but I assure you, you can do it. If you continue to accept despite setback, despite disappointment, despite despair, you will find that gradually the weakness, the panic – all the feelings you dislike so much – will come to mean less and less. As they mean less, they grow less intense, come less often, because they depend on your dislike of them to incite your nerves to bring them. They depend on your dislike of them for their very existence. Utter acceptance removes anxiety, removes bewilderment, removes tension, and so removes the symptoms of stress, and *your symptoms are no more than the usual symptoms of stress*, however unique they may seem to you.

So:

- ✂ Take those first steps at a moderate pace. Do not rush.
- ✂ Realize that you may frighten yourself for some time to come – until habit dies and sensitization improves.
- ✂ Be prepared to think and feel anything. Let come what will.
- ✂ Do not be bluffed by any new, strange, nervous feeling.
- ✂ Accept halts in recovery.
- ✂ Do not waste energy trying to work out why you managed so well one day and so badly the next.
- ✂ Let true acceptance be written on your heart.

The journals (Chapters 9 to 16) give in more detail treatment of many aspects of the anxiety state, including agoraphobia in particular.

CHAPTER 4

Unravelling the Maze
of Nervous Experience

Indecision, suggestibility, loss of confidence, feelings of unreality, of personality disintegration, that dreaded morning feeling, sleeplessness, obsession and depression are described in detail, with their treatment, in my earlier book *Self Help for Your Nerves*. However, these experiences are so important in nervous illness and cause such suffering, confusion and bewilderment, that before I present the journals (Chapters 9 to 16) or continue to talk about agoraphobia, it is necessary to discuss them once more and point out how logically they arise and how simply they can be explained.

INDECISION

Because constant fear and tension have sensitized nerves to produce exaggerated emotions, the slightest change of mind when trying to make a decision can be accompanied by such strong emotional reaction that decision seems impossible. Each point of view appears equally important; right one minute and yet equally wrong the next. Even the simplest decision may seem too much.

A patient once said, 'I used to tie myself in knots thinking: Should I do this or shouldn't I? Whatever I did I worried and thought I shouldn't have done it. Now I act and that's that. Mind you, when I'm in a setback, I go back to the old state of shilly-shally and I can't let the "Whys" drop away easily either!'

He continued, 'Sometimes I say to my wife, "Say something quickly, Mary." This when I'm in such a state I can't make my mind up about anything. Any suggestion Mary makes I cling to.'

Making a decision is especially difficult when the ill person is depleted and at the same time is trying to decide how far he can trust his strength. He doesn't want to overdo things and yet the strain of inactivity is almost impossible to bear. When I discussed this with the same patient, he said, 'That is exactly how I felt a while back. My wife and I went for a run down the coast when I was on holiday, and after we arrived I spent hours trying to decide whether to stay the night or come home. One minute I thought I was too tired to make the journey back, and yet I couldn't bear the thought of staying. As soon as I turned the car round towards home I felt so exhausted at the thought of the trip I was sure we should have stayed. But if we had decided to stay, I know I would have immediately thought we should have gone.'

Thought and feeling so closely tied! Each point of view right one moment and yet equally wrong the next!

SUGGESTIBILITY

A sensitized person can be easily misled into thinking any suggestion which brings such strong reactions as he feels must be important. He becomes suggestible to so much. Reading a newspaper can be a real hazard. A report on illness, especially nervous illness, so impresses him it can upset him for days. He thinks if he hadn't already had all the described symptoms, he soon will have.

A young girl asked me, 'Why do the wrong ideas always come with such force and the right ones seem so shaky?' The wrong suggestions produce fear, and fear is felt so acutely it can over-ride other feelings. It is because the negative, destructive suggestions carry such threat and therefore come with such force that they cling tenaciously and are often mistaken for truth.

The right ideas seem shaky because in a nervous person they have such an insecure foundation; they come only in glimpses. Hope, the feeling the sufferer needs so badly, is so tentative.

LOSS OF CONFIDENCE

Indecision and suggestibility, together with the confusion they bring, must surely lead to loss of confidence. How could they not? Can you see how the pattern unfolds? Such a logical pattern, when we understand how exaggerated emotions can delude us.

The nervous person is not necessarily always without confidence. He can swing from lacking it to being almost elatedly confident. This in itself is confusing. It seems there is no middle of the road for him.

One man, describing his holiday, said, 'It was the last day before coming home. There I was contemplating: Would I go fishing or wouldn't I? I looked at the sea and thought, "No, it's too rough!" It wasn't really rough. I was trying to trick myself. All of a sudden I thought, "I'm going!"

'So out I went on my own and I had the most exhilarating time when I got out there. I caught a lot of fish, and coming in I deliberately let the boat roll about in the sea, and I can remember wading, pushing the boat in front of me with fantastic energy and yet two hours earlier I had been shaking like a jelly at the thought of going.' He paused and said quietly, 'To get over this, you really have to distrust your own mind, haven't you?'

I explained, 'You distrust what it has been saying to you during the years you have been ill. You have good cause. They are the messages that have been keeping you ill. This is why I teach floating past obstructive thought.'

He answered, 'It's like giving yourself the wrong signals. Now you want me to try and give myself the right ones.'

This man was second in charge of an important state industry. So many of my patients, like him, were confident and successful before they became ill and many held responsible positions – teachers, managers, executives. They usually struggled to keep working despite their illness and to do so, while they felt so inadequate and tried to hide their feelings, took great courage.

To regain confidence many needed only insight into the reason for their loss of it and an understanding of sensitization with a programme for desensitization. The return of confidence was automatic, as time and acceptance reduced their symptoms of stress to normal intensity. They were usually relieved to learn that regaining confidence need not be a special objective, that it would return naturally after desensitization.

If nervous illness had been caused by worry which included personal failure of some kind – perhaps dismissal from work – the confidence lost in this way would certainly have to be rebuilt. And, of course, the nervous person who has never been self-reliant finds recovery more difficult, because while he learns how to desensitize himself, he must at the same time build up a confidence he has never had. I discuss this in more detail in Journal 3.

AGITATION

Continuous strain can also bring agitation. After waiting an hour in the Outpatients' Department of a busy psychiatric clinic, many an agitated patient leaves before being seen by the doctor. Of all nervous symptoms, agitation is perhaps the most difficult to bear. It needs urgent relief, and this does mean medication.

UNREALITY

The nervously disturbed person naturally pays more and more attention to what is happening within himself and less and less to outside events. When desperately concerned with our own affairs, it is not easy for any one of us to be interested in a neighbour's new stereo. It is even more difficult for a nervously ill person, whose anxious thoughts are almost compulsively bound within himself. It is this narrowing of interest that leads to a feeling of withdrawal from the outside world, as if there is a veil between it and him, a veil he can neither lift aside nor break through.

'Am I Going Mental, Doctor?'

It is not unusual to hear a patient say, 'I cannot make contact with other people. I feel they're in one world and I'm in another unreal world. It doesn't matter how hard I try, I can't find my way back into their world, the world I used to belong to. Am I going mental, Doctor?' He may have this feeling of unreality in flashes, or it may seem to be always with him.

A nervously ill person can feel unreal in different ways. 'I feel outside myself, watching myself.' Or, 'When I touch things, I know I'm doing it, but can't *feel* I'm doing it.' Another will say, 'It doesn't seem right, or real, to hear somebody laughing.' Happiness has become remote to him because his world of introspection has been full of suffering for so long. Others will say, 'I listen to people talking but half the time I see their mouth move and don't hear what they say. It's like looking at TV with the sound turned off.'

A Feeling Of Unreality Towards Her Daughter

A mother was explaining to me over the telephone how difficult it was for her to accept the feeling of unreality she had towards her daughter. She said that even when she kissed the child good night, she felt she was kissing her in a dream. She explained it was like the feeling she had had when coming out of an anaesthetic.

While we were talking, I heard a commotion in the background. Suddenly, she almost shouted, 'Jessie! For goodness' sake, go outside this minute! I've had just about as much of you this morning as I can stand!' When I pointed out she had just experienced a very real moment of exasperation, she saw my meaning. I showed her she had many real moments with her daughter, but that she was so used to them, they hardly registered. The frightening, unreal moments blotted out the others because she gave them all her attention.

I also pointed out that when she kissed her daughter good night, she always managed to kiss her on the cheek. She didn't kiss the pillow. There was more reality even in that unreal moment than she supposed. She saw the point here also. However, she will need more reassurance to be finally cured. In her present anxious state, her reaction to her own frightening thoughts is so strong that it soon replaces any peace my explanation brings.

Memory Alone Will Bring It

When the cause of feelings of unreality is explained as the natural result of so much anxious introspection, a nervously disturbed person can be so relieved to know he is not going 'mental' he loses his fear. This sudden release could make him feel more real, more part of the outside world, than he has felt for a long time. However this newly gained feeling of reality could be short-lived. His previous experience of feeling unreal is so close, it is only natural that in his sensitized state it will return. Memory along will bring it. And when it comes again, so many make the mistake of being upset and thinking that the cause, for them, must be very deep-seated indeed. A nervously ill person is easily influenced by his feelings of the moment; they are hard to bear and therefore make such an impression that they assume an inflated importance.

So, if a feeling of unreality is part of your suffering, be prepared to work and live with it and accept that for the time being it is natural to feel this way. Feeling unreal is not in the least important and does not mean that you are going 'mental'. With understanding, tension eases and you will gradually find you become less interested in what is happening to you, and more interested in the outside world. You become more outward than inward bound.

OBSESSION

Even obsession fits logically into the pattern and so loses some of its nightmarish quality. Obsession may come when mental fatigue is added to sensitization. Unfortunately few people understand how brain fag works. Frightening thoughts cling and the bewildered sufferer usually makes the mistake of trying to push them away, or to replace them with other thoughts. Occasionally he may be successful, but more often, the more he tries to forget, the more stubbornly the unwelcome ideas cling. As I have said before, discarding thought at will can be difficult, especially when the thought is upsetting and the mind tired. And yet this is what the nervous person so often demands of himself. No wonder he despairs, while he tries desperately to keep unwanted thoughts at bay.

So many obsessions in nervous illness begin this way. They are no more than an unwanted habit established by fear and mental tiredness and, in my experience with my patients, seldom have a deep-seated significance. The nervously ill mother is naturally enough afraid of accidentally harming her child while she is disturbed and lacks confidence and concentration. And she is so suggestible that the thought that she *may* do harm can easily become the fear that she *will*. This does not mean she is aggressive, as some of my patients have been previously told. She is usually no more than a loving but frightened mother with an illness which is following a usual course. This particular fear is shared by many disturbed mothers; surely they could not all be aggressive?

Unfortunately such a woman may be – to her chagrin – convinced she must be peculiar, because as well as fearing she may harm her child she can no longer *feel* love for it or, indeed for any of the family. Actually she is too emotionally drained to register such an uplifting, expansive emotion as love. Everyday emotions depend on vitality for expression and fear may have robbed her of vitality. It is paradoxical that whereas she can feel frightening and unhappy emotions intensely, other emotions seem frozen. She invariably takes this temporary depletion seriously and this adds to her feeling of unreality.

Similarly a nervously ill person may complain of being unable to reach his religion or find comfort in prayer. This can cause havoc to a person dedicated to a religious life.

Thoughts Can Be Grotesque

Thoughts can be grotesque when one is anxious. And the stranger, the more unreal and more frightening they seem the more one may feel compelled to follow them through, almost as if mesmerized, determined to find out the worst.

Whatever your thoughts, however strange, try not to be upset by them. Accept them as normal in your present state, not as something to be dreaded, avoided. Do not make the mistake of supposing there are certain thoughts you must not think, as if there is part of your brain you must not use. Use it all, even the part holding an obsession, and shrink from none of it.

Do not be frightened by your thoughts, however severe the compulsion that may accompany them. Severe tension can give such force to some thoughts that they seem to lock their victim in submission. Even here, *never forget they are only thoughts*, however real and compelling they seem at the moment.

It is the fear, not the thoughts, that tenses, sensitizes, tires. It does not matter how much you dwell on yourself or what you think, if you do not do it fearfully. I am not suggesting one can wipe from one's mind nagging thoughts related to a special problem. When a problem is urgent, the advice to 'Stop worrying and forget about it' is fatuous. The problem must be faced.

FEELINGS OF PERSONALITY
DISINTEGRATION

Surely it is not surprising to hear a nervously ill person say he feels as if his personality is disintegrating, or has disintegrated, when he finds it difficult to make a decision; easy to fall victim to suggestion; difficult to have confidence in himself; when he is bewildered by unreality and perhaps by obsession; and is buffeted by the physical symptoms of stress.

To quote my earlier book, 'He has no inner strength on which to depend; no inner self from which to seek direction … no inner harmony holding thought, feeling and action together.'

Just as confidence returns with desensitization and understanding, so reintegration follows the return of confidence. One does not need to strive for reintegration; one needs to understand and accept apparent disintegration without becoming afraid of or bewildered by it.

None of the experiences discussed (with the exception of obsession) needs separate treatment. To select each and treat it individually is to confuse and complicate. Understanding through explanation – such as given here – can by itself restore inner harmony.

Indecision, suggestibility, loss of confidence, unreality, agitation, personality disintegration and obsession are tiring emotions. The sufferer, harassed by them for months, may gradually deplete his reserves of energy and feel apathetic, depressed. Apathy can be so severe he may have no wish even to bathe himself, much less recover. As part of Journal 6, I discuss nervous depression in detail.

So there is the pattern, beginning with indecision and ending with depression; each stage logically follows the other and each originates from exaggerated emotional reaction to bewilderment and fear. To those who do not understand it, it is often a bewildering maze of one tortured moment after another. And yet, as each stage followed the other to increase suffering, so with enlightenment and acceptance one stage after the other can dissipate into final peace.

THE EVERLASTING WHY? WHY? WHY?

You may think I stress acceptance too much. You may be sceptical about the simplicity of this approach; may have hoped for a more impressive treatment, especially one which does not leave so much for you to do. I stress acceptance because I have seen it cure where all else failed. I have seen it cure people after more than forty years of their trying one different method after another. Indeed, *I have not seen it fail.*

Of course, acceptance is made easier by understanding and this I have tried to give you.

Rising Above A Situation

Consider how acceptance works. It brings a less tense approach; emotions have a chance to calm a little and there is release from asking the everlasting Why? Why? Why? So mental fatigue gradually lifts; the mind becomes more 'flexible'; and when one is no longer confined to one point of view a situation is more easily kept in perspective. This is the meaning of 'rising above a situation'. It is as if the sufferer becomes two people – the first suffering and the second looking on, reconciled to the suffering and also reconciled to trying to accept it. In other words, the second person rises above the suffering.

So, think what you will, but remember to do this with as much acceptance as you can manage, not only up to but *right through* the climax of your fear.

*

CHAPTER 5

Solving the Apparently Insoluble Problem

So far I have talked about people made, and kept, ill by fear of their nervous symptoms rather than by any special problem. However, many people are ill because of some overwhelming problem, sorrow, guilt or disgrace, and I discuss here how an apparently insoluble problem (and this includes sorrow, guilt and disgrace) can cause nervous illness and how one can recover if already made ill in this way.

HOW THE PROBLEM CAUSES ILLNESS

The person who puts himself in danger of nervous breakdown neither solves his problem nor compromises. He spends most of his time dwelling unhappily on the unbearable aspects of his difficulty, torn by indecision and despair. The more anxiously he broods, the tenser he becomes, and because so much constant tension sensitizes his nerves to exaggerate his feelings, his anxiety grows more acute as time passes.

Also, his sensitized nerves may bring the well-known pattern of stress symptoms (churning stomach and so on) and these are so accentuated when he thinks of his problem that concentration on it becomes more and more difficult, decision more elusive, until tension mounts to bring such agitation that the simplest strain can seem unbearable.

Sensitization can exaggerate other emotions as well as anxiety. An event formerly thought sad may now seem tragic. A nervously ill medical student, on duty in the Outpatients' Department, hearing an old woman coughing – with no more than chronic bronchitis – was so moved, he wondered how he would find the fortitude to continue practising medicine.

Such experiences are exhausting, so that there may be little energy left for interest in work, and even in living itself. The sufferer is bewildered by this change within himself and tries hard to get back to being the person he used to be.

So far then, by constant anxious brooding on an apparently insoluble problem, the sufferer has sensitized his nerves to bring upsetting bodily symptoms that frighten him, exaggerated emotions that perplex him, agitation that disturbs him, and all this may finally so exhaust him that he becomes apathetic and depressed.

In addition, constant anxious brooding may gradually slow down thinking until thoughts come haltingly. Also, a tired mind has a tendency to revert continuously to one theme. Whereas in the beginning the sufferer could at will dismiss thinking about his problem, now, because of brainfag, it may seem impossible to forget it, even for a moment.

The inability to think freely makes it increasingly difficult for him to consider his problem flexibly, from different points of view. By now he is able to see it only from one disturbing aspect he has been holding constantly before his eyes during the last months. Indeed, when he thinks of his problem this upsetting point of view may strike so forcibly that he feels completely submerged by it.

Feeling no longer in control of his thoughts or emotions, he sometimes thinks he is going mad. He will clutch desperately at every moment when he feels normal; for example, at times when watching television with the family, he may suddenly feel at peace and think, 'This me at last! If I can stay like this, I'll be all right!' and he clings to such moments, afraid to let them go, for fear that if he loses them he will lose himself.

For a while, after such an experience, he may feel safe, calm. However, because his anxiety has been so intense during the past months, he has only to be anxious once more – which is inevitable in the circumstances – and his reactions will be just as alarming as ever. They must be. His sensitized nerves are triggered to make them so. Naturally, when he panics again, he tries yet harder to grasp outside familiar things to steady himself, to contact reality, to reassure himself all is well. His spirits rise one minute but fall the next. He is now afraid and bewildered *by the state he is in* and still has to cope with the original problem. Indeed, he may now be as much concerned with the way he feels as with the problem itself.

Surely this description shows how constant anxious brooding, when accompanied by lack of understanding and fear, can bring nervous illness, because by now this person is undoubtedly nervously ill.

RECOVERY

To recover, the person made ill by some apparently insoluble problem must first understand that sensitized nerves can exaggerate both emotions and physical symptoms of stress – tears come too readily; laughter may be hysterical; the heart races; the stomach churns. He must then understand the tricks brain fag can play by slowing down thinking and grooving thoughts in a compulsive way. Above all, he must follow understanding with acceptance. He can help calm himself temporarily by using tranquillizers prescribed by his doctor, but must give himself the best tranquillizer of all, understanding and acceptance.

He must be prepared to think as slowly as his tired mind allows and not panic because he cannot think clearly, or because he forgets easily. He must not grasp tensely, fearfully, at those moments when he feels normal, afraid to release them for fear of never contacting them again. He must be prepared to let them come, let them go, as they will. Acceptance releases some tension, enough to begin desensitization. When this happens he is no longer so much at the mercy of his physical reactions and can look at his problem more calmly, more rationally and by degrees give it all his attention.

He Must Find A New Point Of View

Since he has made himself ill by so much brooding on his problem, we may assume no satisfactory action could have been taken, otherwise surely he would have taken it. If no action is possible, he must find a less painful way of looking at the situation. *He must find a new point of view.*

A nervously ill person can rarely do this unaided because, as already mention, his way of thinking has become conditioned by his tense concentration. Every time he thinks of his problem, the established upsetting way of looking at it projects itself immediately and interferes with balance, calm, reasoning. As I said in my earlier book *Self Help for Your Nerves*, he needs a wise counsellor, whether it be doctor, religious adviser, or friend to review the problem dispassionately and help him find a viewpoint which will at least bring some peace. A different way of looking at the problem acts like a crutch for his tired mind. This new approach may not be entirely to his liking, but it must to some extent satisfy him. Peace of mind cannot be forced; so, it is essential the new point of view bring a minimum of pain and fear. A wise counsellor will see to this. A wise counsellor will also need patience, because the nervously ill person may be so mentally tired he could find it difficult to hold the new viewpoint for long. He may see it clearly while discussing it, but may quickly lose his grasp on it when alone and have to discuss the new approach with his adviser many times before he can accept it as his own.

If he can glimpse the new point of view for a few moments each day he will have made a beginning. Indeed, this is the beginning. Although he may repeatedly lose that glimpse and often despair, if he perseveres the glimpse will gradually grow clearer, steadier, last longer, until it becomes the established compromise to bring peace at last.

How Glimpsing Works

A man or woman with high blood pressure may be obsessed with worry about it and continually dwell on the thought of a stroke. Sometimes such a person will say, 'I almost wish the wretched thing would come and get it over!' A person with such worry needs repeated assurance and help in learning how to glimpse, and here tape recordings of consultations are helpful.

First, every practical explanation to allay fear should be given. For example, it should be explained to the sufferer that most of the symptoms a layman thinks are due to high blood pressure usually are not. It is possible to have a pressure so high that, in medical language, it is 'off the machine', and yet feel no symptoms. The headaches familiarly thought due to blood pressure are more often caused by nervous tension than by the pressure itself. Giddiness can be caused by a sudden fall in blood pressure and is not a sign of an impending stroke.

Having reassured him about his symptoms I point out that, though some insurance companies put a high premium on high blood pressure, most people live for years with it. One patient, whose pressure was high at seventy, died at ninety-seven from pneumonia. So a sufferer should understand that he could live many years with his pressure, especially if helped by the advanced treatment of today, and that he could eventually die from some other complaint.

Living with a fear of high blood pressure may take a lot of adjustment – glimpsing – these days, when a layman is subjected to such a barrage from well-intentioned but sometimes misinformed pseudo-medical articles in magazines and newspapers. On some days a patient will come into my surgery happy because he has the right point of view well in focus. On other days, after reading one of these articles, his focus will have slipped and he will be depressed again. However, if he persists in practising glimpsing the right attitude, he eventually becomes philosophical enough to take his 'pressure tablets' without worrying any more than any of us would, and naturally his physical condition benefits.

At first, glimpsing another approach to some difficult problem may seem impossible, because the nervous person feels pulled so strongly towards the old point of view. Also, many different aspects of a problem may disturb; indeed there could be several different problems. Once a person is sensitized, dormant problems can raise their heads and he may successfully glimpse one aspect only to find himself immediately grappling with another. Different aspects occur almost in rotation, like a wheel continually turning. However, if he persists, even this tempestuous experience will pass and he will find he has finally steered himself into calmer waters.

In Journal 4 a woman wrote, 'I found after a week or two, each different fear would fade a little; but I knew my mind had to go through the lot over and over until they finally extinguished themselves. I know this is what you call glimpsing.'

To cope with an apparently insoluble problem:

- Understand and try not to be so upset by physical nervous symptoms, or by exaggerated emotional reaction.
- Try not to be upset if constant brooding slows down thinking, grooves thought, affects memory.
- In addition, one should practise glimpsing the problem from a different point of view.

*

CHAPTER 6

Do – Don't Just Think About Doing

You may often need encouragement and, most important of all, may need to be shown where you continue to make the mistakes holding up progress. These mistakes so often are:

1. You accept 99 per cent of your symptoms and experiences, but withdraw from the final 1 per cent.
2. You let setback throw you into complete despair.
3. You are so paralysed by thinking about doing, you put off the actual doing.

ACCEPTING 99 PER CENT

I have explained so often how acceptance works by gradually reducing the tension that is keeping nerves sensitized; how sensitized nerves magnify ordinary emotions and stress symptoms. I have explained how, even with complete acceptance, it takes time for sensitized nerves to heal and finally record emotions at normal intensity. You may have understood it and set out to practise what I have taught you, but may have found the actual doing so much harder than it seemed when reading about it, or listening to my cassettes.* Why? *Because during the critical moment of greatest suffering you withdrew; you recoiled.*

When you tensely withdrew, your body released more adrenalin, more stress hormone, which increased sensitization, so you instinctively sought relief by running away from the situation.

The next time you set off to practise acceptance, and I am not talking only about agoraphobia, *watch for the moment of recoil and go towards it* in a loose, floating kind of way. That is the key.

An air-pilot recently explained that the same principle held in his work. When a plane is going into a fall – a ground loop – one of the hardest lessons for a beginner to learn is to head the plane into the direction of the fall and not try to recover balance by tipping the wings in the opposite direction. To draw away like this is fatal; to go towards is to flatten out and recover balance.

To choose a more common experience. Those who ride a bicycle know that if, when about to fall, they turn the wheel in the direction of the fall, the bicycle rights itself; if they turn it in the opposite direction – as beginners invariably do – they fall.

You may fail in the beginning, perhaps often, but you will eventually succeed if you recognize the old enemy *withdrawal* and do not let it take charge of the situation, as you have been doing. *Watch that last 1 per cent.* Passing through that last 1 per cent can turn part acceptance into full acceptance and cure. Never forget : *you make your own crisis by withdrawal.*

* For a full list of Dr Weekes' cassettes and recordings, and information on where to obtain them, see p. 425.

🎄 Peace lies on the other side of panic.

🎄 Withdrawal is your jailer.

🎄 Pass through that last 1 per cent.

ON NOT LETTING A SETBACK
THROW YOU

Being bogged down by setback is another form of withdrawal. Memory is always ready to defeat you by reminding you of so many other defeats. However far you may sink into setback, never lose the desire to go forward again to recovery. Do not be put off by the places and experiences you fear. These are your salvation, *because recovery lies in such places, such experiences.*

What Is Recovery?

Recovery is the final establishment of the right attitude of mind. You can practise thinking the right way, however deep you may find yourself in setback. It is difficult to switch from despair to quiet, determined hope, *but you can do it.*

Thousands have despaired as you have and yet have changed their attitude to finally recover. You have as much courage as they. Courage is not given to one and denied another. The difference is that some draw on the courage given, others do not. Courage has never failed to come to those who really want it. The secret lies in that *really*. So do not let any setback bluff you into refusing to practise again.

Also, do not be disappointed if the symptoms and fears coming in setback stay acute for a while, even when you truly accept them. When you resensitize yourself by being afraid of setback, more time must be allowed for this added sensitization to heal, and for your slight grip on hope to firm again. In the beginning, it is as if each setback must run a certain prescribed course before it spends itself. Accept this also.

⚹ Recovery lies in the places you fear.
⚹ Seek them with utter acceptance.

PARALYSIS BY CONTEMPLATION

You may shrink from the thought of recovery in the future and the demands this may bring. You imagine meeting those demands as you feel now – ill. Let me remind you again, recovery brings its own change. It brings renewed strength, renewed interest, and with these comes ability to cope. Go forward with trust in this change; trust in a gradual merging into normal living. It is the gradualness that makes all possible. But it is this very gradualness that is so hard to bear, because it is so frustrating. Also gradualness allows so much time for contemplation, and during the early stages of recovery *contemplation is the killer*. Over such a long time, imagination has added so many difficulties to recovering that these have come to seem too real, too concrete to be talked away, thought away by you. Only repeated doing will iron them out; *only repeated doing will take the fear out of contemplation*.

My words can only show the way. Also your understanding is still possible only in thought. Feeling it in your heart as certainty is another matter and experience along can put certainty in your heart. Your experience of success has been so slight so far, you have probably only occasionally glimpsed it. This is hard to bear, because it makes you impatient to grasp and hold what you have glimpsed, and patience is never a nervous person's strong point.

So do not be disheartened if, at this stage, you simply cannot see yourself doing this or that. The thought of it may seem a hopeless dream. And yet salvation lies in repeated doing. It lies in doing until the habit of doing is so well established it replaces the habit of defeatist thinking. This takes time and effort. The habit of defeatist thinking is so strong that although you may have made many successful journeys, accomplished many difficult tasks, deciding to try again may sometimes seem as difficult as ever. Try not be be disturbed by this. Let more time pass, until more and more achievement accumulates to bring finally the certainty you crave.

You Can't Postpone The School Meeting

So, do not wait for the best moment to make that special effort. The school meeting on the 15th may come at a particularly bad moment for you, but you cannot postpone the school meeting. The more often you practise my teaching when you do not feel your best, the more confident you will gradually become to face anything at any time, however you may feel. This is the only way to make an appointment or any future undertaking seem less menacing. *Wait on no mood*. It's the sitting waiting, hat and coat on, clutching handbag, contemplating moving that is so devastating. Don't let contemplation shackle you. You can still succeed, however 'bad' you feel before the actual time of 'doing'. The confidence you gain by succeeding when you feel your worst is the most invaluable, enduring, dependable confidence of all.

- ✤ Recovery brings its own strength.
- ✤ Only repeated doing takes fear out of contemplation.
- ✤ Salvation lies in repeated doing.
- ✤ Wait on no mood.

✻

CHAPTER 7

Taking the First Steps

When first reading this book, you may feel encouraged to practise as advised and yet may be afraid to take the first step. If you
are afraid in this way, it is usually for one or more of the reasons
mentioned at the beginning of the book:

1. You have been ill so long you think you are beyond help.
2. You do not trust yourself to try again. You have tried so many
    different ways to recover in the past and have – as you think
    – let yourself down so badly you haven't the heart to begin
    again.
3. You understand what I advise, but you panic so easily that,
    despite your best efforts, you seem to wilt before each
    onslaught.
4. You feel so emotionally, mentally and physically weary you
    shrink from taking the first step. That first step opens up
    such a vista of effort, you quail before it.

YOU THINK YOU HAVE BEEN ILL
TOO LONG TO RECOVER

First, understand no outside force is doing this to you. Your body is simply responding to the way you think. It may be sensitized, but although sensitization seems to come from the depths of your being, it is really superficial and can be healed. This healing power is in each of us. You have it as much as anyone else; you are simply standing in its way. Your body is not irrevocably altered physiologically by your illness. If you have been ill for years (and I have known people nervously disturbed for most of their life), it means only that the habit of nervous illness will be strongly entrenched and memory discouraging. But you have the power to accept and discount these barriers to recovery. You still have the power of freewill *through acceptance*, although it may seem as if you have not. You have it.

However, although a nervously ill person may find peace and understanding while with his doctor, he may have forgotten most of the good advice a few hours later because his tired mind forgets so easily. This makes taking the first steps especially difficult. Hence, for my patients I record an interview to encourage taking first steps, to encourage the act of getting moving. Just as the nervous person has bombarded himself with defeatist suggestions over the past months, now he can bombard himself with a doctor's constructive advice on a tape recording (or LP records* if a tape is not available), until it becomes so much part of himself he *feels* its meaning strongly enough to find the courage to set off. I stress again: there is, in my opinion and experience, no such thing as a chronic anxiety state which

---

* For a full list of Dr Weekes' cassettes and recordings, and information on where to obtain them, see p. 425.

cannot be cured if the sufferer understands what is needed of him and is willing to play his part.

YOU DO NOT TRUST YOURSELF

It doesn't matter if you don't trust yourself. I am not asking you to. I ask you only to try to understand the advice I give and trust *it*. However big a coward you may think yourself now, *the advice still works*. You do not have to cure yourself; you let your body do that. You simply stand aside, out of the way, by adding as little *second* fear as possible – resisting adding 'Oh, my goodness' and 'What if?' Trust your body to heal itself while you practise the teaching here. It has responded faithfully to the wrong messages you have been sending it; it will respond just as faithfully to the right ones – although more reluctantly at first.

YOU UNDERSTAND, BUT FEAR FLASHES SO FIERCELY YOU WILT BEFORE IT

You may have to accept much flashing fear for the time being. You probably feel that when panic strikes you cannot think at all; so that practising 'going with it' seems impossible. However severe the panic, if you watch yourself closely you will discover that you can think, even if the wrong thoughts. Practising going with, and not shrinking from, fear is like learning to ride a bicycle. There is a certain amount of falling off before you finally learn to ride. But unless you pick yourself each time and try again, you never learn. Never forget that *failure is not finality*.

To teach a patient a practical way to meet his fear, I press my hand hard against his chest and ask him to move forward against the pressure. As he strains forward, I point out that this is the tense way he has been reacting to fear. I then ask him to stretch his arms out before him, and move them as if swimming forward in deep, cool water. Usually, I can feel some of the tension relax immediately.

Some people so dislike the thought of water, they avoid bathing; even avoid washing their hair. To them I suggest the feeling of drifting forward on a cloud. This, or thinking of swimming forward in deep, cool water, is not as foolish as it may sound. It brings a feeling of release and gives something positive and helpful to do at a critical moment when otherwise one would probably withdraw tensely in defeat. So when you take those first steps, take them 'in deep, cool water' or in any other relaxed way (floating forward) you care to imagine.

YOU THINK YOU HAVEN'T THE STRENGTH TO TAKE THAT FIRST STEP

In my earlier book, I described a woman who, 'exhausted' by her nerves, had been more or less confined to a couch for months, believing she was too weak to stand for long. As treatment, I urged her to begin painting the woodwork on the back porch. Against her will, and to her husband's amazement, she began. In a few days she was painting with interest.

So much nervous weakness is encouraged by loss of confidence in what one's body can do. Remember this weakness is not true organic, muscular weakness, although it may feel like it; so don't let it keep you on a couch. Your muscles grow stronger only as you use them. Once more I stress that you should be examined by your doctor and assured your weakness is nervous.

If you have the slightest urge to practise what I advise, encourage it by making the effort to take that first step:

- ✞ however long you may have been ill;
- ✞ however much you may distrust yourself;
- ✞ however afraid you may be;
- ✞ however tired you think you are.

❧

CHAPTER 8

A Husband's Attitude to his Wife's Illness

I had just spent an hour with a sick woman. It was essential that I speak to her husband, and I found him polishing his car in the driveway. He continued polishing as I spoke and did not raise his eyes. After I had given him a full explanation of his wife's condition and asked for his co-operation, he blurted out, 'Mashed potato! Always mashed potato! Why not chipped potatoes?'

I explained as patiently as I could that his wife could not cope with three small children and chipped potatoes at the same time.

He was not convinced. 'How much longer will she be like this?' If she would stop swallowing all those pills and pull up her socks, she would be all right! He knew plenty of women with more children than his wife, and they weren't like this. This was stupid. This wasn't the girl he married. How soon would she again be the girl he married?

This man did not mean to be cruel to his wife. He simply did not understand. Nervous illness is so bewildering. Doctors disagree about cause and treatment, so it is small wonder that husbands are perplexed. In the beginning this man sympathized with his wife, but when the illness dragged on, while all the time his wife looked well enough, talked sensibly enough, he found it more and more difficult to remain patient. It seemed so silly to him that a woman of her age should be afraid to go shopping on her own. He would look at her in amazement, unable to understand how a woman who had taken a 'big operation' without a murmur could now be afraid to go out without him. To mention going to the movies was enough to send her into a panic. When he asked why, she would answer only 'I'm too frightened!' This was no explanation from a grown woman.

It was difficult for her to explain to a man 'without a nerve in his body' how, while she waited in a line at the shop, the tension would mount until it seemed unbearable and she would feel urged to run outside before she fainted or 'something terrible' happened. Small wonder the husband was confused when she returned without the food she had gone to buy. Surely it is not hard to understand why this man went on polishing his car, truculently demanding chipped potatoes. To him, home cooked chips meant normal living. No wonder he wanted her to stop all this nonsense.

Alas! no one wanted this more than she, but finding a way to stop the nonsense meant finding her way to recovery, and until recently this had seemed beyond her.

It is not easy for a doctor to tell a man, harassed by an emotionally distressed wife, disturbed children, and household bills that his wife's quick recovery depends so much on his continued patience and that he must try to understand even when understanding seems hard, so that he will add as little tension as possible to his wife's suffering.

A wife will say, 'When I try to explain to my husband, Doctor, I can see by the look on his face that he thinks I'm crazy or something. It's not his fault. But I wish he wouldn't go to pieces so quickly when he sees me like this. I wish he wouldn't think he's helping me by trying to force me to do things. It's when he does this that the tension mounts, and that's what frightens me so much, Doctor.'

A HUSBAND NEEDS ENCOURAGEMENT

A husband's co-operation is so important that a doctor should explain as fully to him as to his wife what is happening and how she can be cured. A husband needs explanation, encouragement and support, so that his criticism can be turned into constructive help. The added tension of being watched by a pair of critical eyes helps keep a wife in a cycle of tension-worry-tension.

The husband has but to go off in a huff in the morning to throw his wife into despair for the day. He may forget about it until he reaches for his hat when his work is over, but she has been 'with it' since he left. And you may be sure that, in his desperate state (and his is a desperate state), he delivered a few telling broadsides before leaving, especially that final thrust, as he closed the door, about the cross he bears. The woman, left alone with perhaps only children for company, or with no company at all, now has not only her cross to carry, but his as well.

BACK ON THE SAME OLD RAZZLE-DAZZLE

Of course she tries to talk sense to herself. Part of her trouble is arguing with herself and getting nowhere. One minute she decides to stop all this nonsense once and for all, to let none of it get her down; the next moment she's at it again, back on the same old razzle-dazzle, back with 'Oh, my goodness' and 'What if ...?'

The entire day is a battlefield strewn with good resolves and as many failures. No wonder she is confused and afraid of what is happening to her. She asks why everything should seem so impossible. If only her husband could understand how trapped she feels, how desperately she wants to be her old self again. If only he could understand that his inability to stay the course with his wife, his pressing urgency for her to recover, his tendency to belittle her illness, are some of the main reasons for her delayed recovery.

CASSETTES AND VIDEO

It may be difficult, even impossible, to persuade a husband to read this book. Here my cassettes have a special mission. Many reluctant husbands find themselves listening despite themselves. Even disapproving relatives will listen to cassettes or watch a video, and it can be gratifying to the sufferer to hear someone say later, 'Now, I understand at last.'

ALL CHILDREN, FOOD, CHORES

Some aspects of housekeeping can hardly be called interesting, especially preparing food for children and trying to force it down reluctant throats or scraping it off the floor after losing the battle. The average mother puts up with this when well, because she mixes it with happier experiences. When nervously ill nothing may interest her. Life becomes all children, food, chores, and this adds to her confusion because *it used not to worry her like this*.

In nervous illness emotions are so grossly exaggerated that mild dislikes may become revulsions, and it may seem impossible for the mother to change them back into mild dislikes so that she can tolerate them again.

Some husbands withdraw from the situation. They've 'had it' and find refuge away from home. Friends may not help. 'Poor George! I don't know how you have put up with it for so long!' may be handed to George with a friendly drink, and if George hadn't already wondered himself, he certainly does now.

THE END OF HER TETHER

It is difficult to convince a man how much his wife's recovery may depend on him. It is a difficult task to say to a man, almost as exhausted as his wife, 'However upset you are, however strained your patience, your nerves, you must try to be patient a little longer. If you are at the end of your tether, what about your wife? She saw the end of her tether months ago and she is still trying. Don't make her feel that everything depends on her quick recovery. That is too much for a sick woman to bear.'

If a husband takes the trouble to try to understand and help, his reward will be the grateful, deep love of a wife who will never forget his strength, kindness, and dependability in her illness. If he does not, despite the many excuses she will make for him she will find it hard to forget that he failed her when she needed him most, and her illness may drag on unnecessarily.

Essential Help for Your Nerves

The Journals

Presenting eight quarterly journals based on those written during 1968–70 for 1,300 sufferers from nervous illness in the British Isles, the United States of America, Canada, Australia, New Zealand, South Africa, Hong Kong, India and recently Japan.

As these journals were written at quarterly intervals, each reader had three months between issues in which to assimilate and practise the teaching. It may help the present reader to know this, so that he does not expect too much from himself in one reading.

✤

CHAPTER 9

Journal 1

Why Recovery Seems so Difficult
to so many Nervously Ill People

A nervously ill person needs one set plan for recovery, and should not be pulled one way and another by considering different methods of treatment; torn by indecision whether he is on the right track or not; whether he should try this or that. Because I understand how confused you can so quickly become in this way, I want to keep in touch with you, and encourage you through your moments of discouragement and despair.

Do not think that because I am sending quarterly journals I believe you will take a long time to recover. I know how suggestible your illness makes you, and how easily you could jump to this conclusion. Some of you have trodden such well-worn tracks of misery for so many years that recovery may indeed be slow; but there are many who, through book and records, are already on the way to recovery, and who will certainly not be needing much longer the advice I will give in these bulletins.

However, even when recovered (how good that sounds), some may be interested to read the journal, whenever it may come.

WHY RECOVERY SEEMS SO DIFFICULT TO THE NERVOUSLY ILL

By nervously ill, I mean people who suffer from excessive anxiety, panic, fears and upsetting physical nervous symptoms. In other words, people who have been examined by their doctor and told they are suffering from 'nerves'.

Before beginning, I would like you to understand I realize I am talking to a mixed group of people – to young, middle-aged, old; to men and women; some ill for a long time, some for a short time; some with special problems, some agoraphobic, others not agoraphobic. I assure you I will bear this in mind and will endeavour to include something in each talk for each of you.

I am now sorting the hundreds of application forms for journals you have sent me, and noting your different kinds of fears. Knowing how susceptible you are to suggestion, I will be very careful how I speak about these fears. There will be nothing frightening in these journals, I assure you.

Agoraphobia

First, the word 'agoraphobia': it simply means fear of travelling far from home; fear of being where help cannot be had quickly; loss of confidence in being able to manage one's reactions in crowded places, and so on. Agoraphobia is only one of the many aspects of nervous illness. Isn't it natural that people already nervously ill who have weak 'turns' when out should eventually avoid going out? Of course it is. And once they do this, they could be called agoraphobic.

Personally I do not like labels and rarely mention the word agoraphobia to my patients. Defined in this way it assumes unwarranted specialization and so seems to take on unnecessary importance. It is no more than one phase of a general anxiety state. I wish to assure you it is curable, labelled or not. Do not be depressed by anything you may read, or hear, to the contrary. So much depends on the person treating it, as well as on the person seeking cure. I have seen many patients cured after more years of suffering than some of you may have lived. So cheer up!

Problems

Those of you with special problems may think, 'All this is very well, but Dr Weekes can't help me with my particular problems.' I may not be able to help you with your individual problems – limited as I am to contacting you through journals alone – but I can show you certain general aspects of recovery that will help you. For example, in addition to being upset by your special problems, worrying about them too much and for too long brings its own emotional and physical suffering which is common to all who suffer as you do. By helping you understand and cope with this, I will at least be able to relieve you of part of your burden and so enable you to approach your problems more whole-mindedly and perhaps not be so overcome by them.

The Night At The Local

A nervously ill person is not easy to live with, and in time a once sympathetic family may begin to react unsympathetically – the husband becoming almost as 'nervy' as the sick wife, so that he may take to staying late at night at the 'local'. He may also start harassing his wife to 'snap out of it', trying to push her, hurry her forward to recovery. Tension builds up between them and gradually makes the old companionship become a dependency on the part of the wife, and this is a torture to her, an exasperation to the husband. Relationships with the in-laws may become strained, even relationships with one's own parents, brothers, sisters.

With recovery, these difficulties ease; so try not to be too depressed by them now. It is ironic that some of the problems helping to keep you ill would not be there if you were not ill. They are encouraged by the state you are now in, although you may not recognize this. They automatically resolve themselves as you recover.

Do You Know What Recovery Really Means?

When most nervous people think of recovery, *they imagine a completely peaceful body* and think that while their body continues to bring any nervous symptoms they must still be ill, that their reactions are sick reactions and would not be there if they were well.

Let us be quite clear about this. The monsters that plague the nervously ill person's life are the usual reactions to stress any of us may feel from time to time. They plague the nervous person because they are exaggerated by his sensitization – not simply because they are present. *It is the exaggeration that is the sickness, not the presence.* Let me illustrate this.

Suppose you hear a high pitched sound. It is not nice, but not so very disagreeable, so you go on working. Intensify this sound until it becomes extremely loud, and it may then seem so unbearable it prevents your working. *Yet it is the same sound, only louder*. So it is with the physical sensations of nervous illness. They are the same normal reactions we all feel to any stress that may come during our day, but to the nervously ill, sensitized person they are so much, shall we say, louder, they may seem almost unbearable.

Recovery lies, not in completely ridding oneself of these reactions – as so many believe – but in *reducing them to normal intensity and normal frequency*. To achieve 'normal frequency' means being able to quieten one's body so that nervous responses do not come at every provocation, as they do now – at a thought, an anxious memory. It means creating some insulation between you and stress.

Normal Reaction Is Tricking Him

The nervously ill person is blinded to the road to recovery because he does not recognise the basis of normality in his strange feelings.

This is one of the main reasons why he feels lost. He goes round in circles trying to rid himself of something that is normal in the circumstances; something that, in a milder form, must always be part of his daily life while he is alive. He would have to be anaesthetized, unconscious, sound asleep, to feel no stress, and so be rid of all nervous symptoms!

Even those not nervously ill must have some variation in their normal daily nervous reactions. For example, on some days reaction to any stress will seem more severe than on others. Of course, this natural variation also comes to the nervously sick person. But does he accept it as normal? To be expected? Not he! The days when his reactions are more severe, he thinks he must be more ill, and thrashes himself with added despair and depression. Normal variation in daily nervous reaction is another puzzling pitfall on the way to recovery, and it is a pitfall which never fails to trap a sick person into trying to find a reason for it.

It May Be So Long Since He Was Well

All this is understandable, because it may be so long since the nervously ill person was well that he may have forgotten what it felt like to be well. He has forgotten the natural nervous reactions he had then, because they did not bother him. He accepted them as part of his day, even expected them. At some time or other when he was well most variations had occurred; even the palpitations on running up stairs, the churning stomach before asking his boss for a rise, or before sitting for an examination.

Because he fails to see this basis of normality in the nervous reactions he has now, he is misled into struggling to throw them off completely, or into trying to stop them coming. No one can completely throw off normal reactions, especially when they are exaggerated. So, he is tricked into trying to do the impossible. Is it any wonder recovery seems so difficult to so many nervously ill people?

Three First-Class 'A' Levels

Here is a practical example. Suppose after much sacrifice on her part, a mother hears her son has gained three first-class 'A' levels. When she first hears the news might her heart not pound a little, beat faster? Her hands tremble? Might she not break out into a sweat, her face flush – leave her lunch untouched because her excitement has taken away her appetite, be breathless, go 'weak all over' and have to sit down for a while? Surely each of these feelings taken separately could be described as unpleasant, and yet she feels them as part of happiness. Her interest is so firmly fixed on her son's success, she hardly notices what is happening to her physically. Her inner feeling of joy is so acute that the stressful symptoms that accompany it all seem part of it and therefore easy to bear.

Also, she knows that in a little while her reactions will settle down; even if she has had 'quite a turn' it will soon pass. So, she waits contentedly without worrying about its passing, and, of course, the feelings gradually calm.

May I remind you again these feelings of happy stress are the same feelings that come with nervous illness? They differ only in being less severe and in being accompanied by a different emotional tone.

In Place Of Happiness Put Panic

In place of a happy incident put an impending visit by a nervously ill woman to the hairdresser, dentist or school meeting. Instead of happiness, she feels an inner core of apprehension, even panic, and whereas the happy woman did not worry about her stress symptoms, the nervously ill woman notices her feelings immediately because:

1. They have been coming so consistently, for such a long time, that they are triggered to come more acutely than the feelings of stress that accompany the shock of unexpected happiness.
2. They are so well known to the nervously ill person, that she anticipates them – even goes looking for them – with feelings of dread, fear.
3. When in fear, thoughts are invariably turned inward, not outward as in happiness; so she becomes even more conscious of what is happening within herself than of outside

events. Palpitations are always unpleasant, but do they really upset when the heart palpitates for joy? Consider that.

An Ordinary Day In a Nervously Ill Housewife's Life

Since the majority of my nervously ill patients have been housewives who are alone all day (how little some husbands understand what this means), perhaps with one or two children dragging at her skirt, I will describe the day of a nervously ill housewife and show how she holds back her own recovery by trying to rid herself of her reactions. Do not think I have forgotten the lonely spinster, the bachelor, or the married man who struggles to work each day. Fundamentally they will find their situation and their reactions are not so different from those of the housewife. At least, it will not be difficult for them to substitute their situation for hers, and to apply my explanation to themselves.

Waking Up

On first waking in the morning, realization that another day is here to be faced may strike the sick housewife before she even opens her eyes. This thought immediately brings anguish, and anguish reawakens the symptoms of stress. Then as she wakens further, and remembers more vividly some threatening duty of the day – perhaps a school function at night, or Wednesday's heavy midweek shopping – more spasms of anguish follow, one after the other, so the sensations she dreads finally merge into one long, inner churning. To her this is a very disappointing start to the day and a very tiring one.

After further panic, with her resistance already lowered by months, years of suffering, she may feel exhausted and then depressed. What little store of energy she has gained from her night's rest is almost depleted by nervous reaction to her own thoughts even before she tries to get herself out of bed. Her limbs seem so leaden she may feel incapable of moving them. However, necessity eventually forces her up and she finally 'points the body' (as one woman put it) at the day's work.

Now she is fumbling under the bed for her slippers. The very repetition of stooping and groping under the bed and then forcing her foot past that faded nylon pompom brings back the memory of the countless mornings she has done the very same thing feeling exactly as she does now. Memory, what misery you can bring when we let ourselves be driven by you! Unhappy memory and despair are cousins, so this housewife sighs deeply in despair as she struggles into her dressing gown. Trapped by memory, her thoughts become all despair, and since her body is at the mercy of her thoughts, what else can it do but feel 'worse than ever'! *She has already made memory part of the day's burden* – a big mistake.

She used not to feel like this. Indeed, she may have been active and most capable. Feeling this way is so unlike her old self it seems as if she is two people, one moving in a dream, the other getting breakfast. She feels unreal.

The Sudden Silence Seems Overpowering

When the noise of the family's departure is abruptly stilled by the final closure of the front door, the sudden silence seems more overpowering than the noise had been. At least the noise meant someone was there – a prop to help divert attention. Now all that attention is directed to herself and the last thing she wants is to have her mind on herself, on her illness. And yet she knows this is exactly what she will have, probably for the whole day. There seems no way out for her. Her heart quails at the thought. Whose wouldn't? More anguish. So, as she pours herself a cup of tea before facing the stack of dishes in the sink, she thinks how hopeless it all is, how futile to imagine she could possibly recover, when she can hardly find the strength, or courage, to face one day.

Is it any wonder she feels defeated? Look at the circle in which she has been turning, almost like the blindfolded ass that drags the millstone round and round to grind the corn. Look at the circle ... memory of past suffering and the anticipated suffering of the day ahead bring despair ... despair brings stress ... stress brings even more acutely sensitized feelings ... which lead to more despair. And the cycle continues, back to more stress and so on.

What a pattern! And this pattern is repeated in so many of the day's activities. Consider the shopping. This housewife may not leave the house to go shopping until mid-morning, and between waking and setting off she gives herself little spurts of panic whenever she thinks of the outing to come. Two hours of intermittent panic would weaken even a strong man, so by the time mid-morning comes her legs already feel weak and wobbly and she feels light-headed, giddy. She is not surprised by this. She has been expecting and dreading it. It is one of the reasons why she doesn't want to go out alone. She thinks it is part of her illness, and to avoid feeling this way while out she would rather not go. She had hoped today might be different, but once again she thinks she will be forced to send the children to do the shopping, when they return from school.

At the thought of school, her heart misses a beat – the school meeting that evening! She had forgotten about that! How will she make *that*, when she feels so weak already? More anguish. And what if they ask her to look at the children's paintings in the crowded, hot classroom! That would be the end! School function – heavens! That means half an hour under the drier at the hairdresser's. She had forgotten that one too! Anguish, more anguish.

So there she is. To every situation – and yet, such ordinary situations – she panics, and her body dutifully and naturally answers with more stress-sensations. She does not understand that these are not sick reactions, that the sickness lies in their exaggeration, not in their actual occurrence.

'Will I? Won't I?'

When she thinks of disappointing the family once more, she feels lost. So, one minute she decides to go, the next minute she cannot face the thought of it. After an hour or so of 'Will I? Won't I? Can I? Can't I?' the tension of indecision brings on agitation; agitation makes her tremble and when this starts she feels utterly defeated.

The sad part of all this is that she has defeated herself. The feelings she dreads most are intense simply because months, years of fear have made them so. For example, her fear of the weakness uses up extra glucose and this creates more weakness. Her fear of panic produces more adrenalin, which excites her nerves to produce more panic; but she is not a doctor and does not understand this. So she stays blindly afraid, blindly weak, blindly at home. Once more she thinks her body is doing this to her. So it is, but by merely responding in a physiologically correct way to the fears she brings it.

The Physiology Of Nervous Weakness

Let me explain the physiology of nervous weakness. To provide energy for movement, our body burns glucose in our muscle cells. Glucose is also burnt for energy to express emotion – fear, anger, even joy. This glucose circulates in our blood. When we use up available supplies of glucose too quickly with too much emotion, there may not be enough to provide energy for normal movement. Although we can still move, we feel weak and shaky. Also, the adrenalin released by stress dilates blood vessels in our muscles, so that blood drains from our body into our legs, adding to our feeling of weakness. If we wait as calmly as possible, our liver will break down its stored glycogen into glucose and liberate this extra supply. In addition, the blood vessels gradually recover their normal tone and blood circulates normally.

But does this woman wait patiently? Even as patiently as her 'nerves' will let her? Not she. She becomes even more agitated by the weakness, and so burns up much of the extra glucose as her liver supplies it. Naturally the weakness takes unnecessarily long to pass.

Of course, it is the thought of what might happen while she is out that is helping to bring the panic. What could happen outside is only a repetition of what has been happening at home since early morning. She has already gone a long way towards suffering as intensely as she could away from home, but does not realize it.

How Can She Face The Drier At The Hairdresser's?

In place of weakness, she may feel stiffness in her legs; they seem difficult to move. This stiffness – sometimes almost a feeling of paralysis – is no more than muscular contraction, a body's normal response to excessive tension. Neck muscles may also be tense; in her words, her neck 'feels awful'. Agitation makes her heart race, her face flush; she feels burning 'all over', as if she will 'burst'. Feeling this way, how can she face the drier at the hairdresser's? How will she manage to sit there 'chained' for half an hour! More panic. And yet, for the sake of a family that cannot possibly measure her sacrifice, this woman may battle into the salon to face a hell her own fears have created in her sensitized body.

Surely these are reasonable fears. None of these experiences is nice to have. Anyone would want to withdraw from them. Yet, they are all normal reactions in the circumstances, and to recover *she must not hope to abolish them but to reduce them to normal intensity*. This is the only answer.

She Dreams The Impossible Dream

Let us return to that early morning awakening and see how she can be helped.

If she expects to wake feeling well at this stage in her illness, she dreams the impossible dream. One night's sleep will not work that miracle. Yet this is exactly what she does expect. Each night when she lays her head on the pillow, she prays for just that – to wake up feeling her old self. Before she even goes to sleep, her very hopes are preparing the way for disappointment the next day; so when she wakens and feels as ill as ever, of course her body registers anguish. It is only reacting naturally to her disappointment. Her body is her servant; it follows her directions, although she may not even put into words what she thinks; may not even think clearly. She may simply *feel* misery and then an overwhelming flood of disappointment follows; and disappointment that is inevitable while her body is as sensitized as it is. Knowing the facts about sensitization as we now know them, surely it is easy to see that her overwhelming flood of disappointment was wasted emotion and an unnecessary drain on her limited resources of strength.

If one could only whisper in her ear ear at night: 'Do not be disappointed, however you feel in the morning. Please do not add despair and exhaust yourself still further. Just for once, be prepared to take yourself as you find yourself without being so upset because you are as you are. Do not knock your head against the brick wall of despair. Play along with it tomorrow to the best of your ability. Try not to expect the impossible now; you will be like this for a while yet, so if you must "point" the body, point it willingly. When you go to bed, do not pray to wake feeling well. *Pray to wake with the courage to accept yourself as you find yourself in the morning.*'

Breaking The Chain Of Memory

When she fumbles under the bed for her slippers, she needs special help. She should buy new slippers for a start – and if possible rather foolish ones, that make her smile – at least a new pair. She might try to remember to put them somewhere else, not under the bed every night. Breaking the chain of memory helps in such foolish little ways as this. It breaks the repetition of moments of suffering, so she does not think despair so readily. When she thinks despairingly, she immediately feels despair. This is a natural reaction in her state. So many of her early morning reactions are to be expected in the circumstances. As already mentioned, *it is the exaggeration in the feeling of despair, the exaggeration in her body's responses, that is the sickness.*

To help herself further she could change the position of the furniture in her room especially the bed, so that on waking she does not see the same familiar pattern of things – that special spot on the ceiling – to remind her of the many other mornings of identical suffering.

'Even If My Legs Go Weak They Can Still Carry Me!'

If only she would give herself a chance during those hours of waiting to go shopping and say to herself, 'If I keep frightening myself of course my legs will feel weak and I'll feel giddy. That's only natural, and it is not an illness. Even if they go weak, they can still carry me when I go out. So I'll try to walk as calmly as I can manage, however I feel. If my legs can carry me home after I've been panicking, surely they can carry me forward in between panics. If I do this as willingly as I can, my liver will supply more glucose and the weakness will gradually pass!'

At last she would be giving her body a chance. If she would continue saying, 'Of course I'll feel awful at the hairdresser's. I've been feeling awful there for so long, I'm not going to stop feeling awful now, just because I want to! I may make great strides doing other things – like going for a holiday – and still find the hairdresser's just as difficult, perhaps worse, when I come home. This doesn't mean I am sick again. It only means memory is up to her old tricks. I will probably have to sit through the hour at the hairdresser's many times thinking the right way before I no longer dread going there!'

You, who are suffering and read this, turn your attention to the way you think, not to your feelings. Come to terms with your attitude and your feelings will look after themselves.

I wish to mention two different kinds of sufferers. One says, 'I can't help any of it coming. It just comes. I'm not doing it to myself. I suddenly feel dreadful when I'm not even thinking about my illness. That is what is so hard to understand.'

The other says, 'I know I am doing this to myself, but I feel powerless to stop it. That is what is so terrible!'

'I Can't Help Any Of It Coming!'

Consider the first person. There are indeed times when some nervous symptoms do seem to strike for no special reason and appear to be unrelated to the sufferer's occupation at that particular moment. However, they are a result of what he has done to himself in the past. Past suffering has prepared nervous reactions to come so swiftly and easily that the slightest stimulus, perhaps unrecognized by him, and certainly beyond his direct control, may bring them. However, it is in his power to gradually soothe this hyper-irritability by accepting these 'out-of-the-blue' attacks and not being continually surprised and upset by them.

'I Am Doing This To Myself'

The person who says he knows he is frightening himself and is powerless to stop it must try to understand this is only a natural outcome of his body's instant response to his slightest thought. As I have pointed out before, in a sensitized person, feeling – especially fear – follows thought so closely, not only do they both often seem as one, but sometimes it seems as if there is no thought – only feeling. This in itself is confusing and hard to bear; so the nervous person stays frightened with no outside cause for his fear. Naturally he thinks he is frightening himself and in a sense he is. His aim should be to reduce the intensity and speed of his responses, so that reason can come into the picture. To do this he must try to look ahead and not stay emotionally bound to each minute of the day. He needs a long-range programme. Let him say to himself, 'I've been frightening myself for a long time, I'll probably go on doing it while my feelings respond so quickly to what I am thinking. If I understand this is because I am sensitized, and if I try not to be too

292   *Essential Help for Your Nerves*

upset by it, then perhaps in a little while fear may not come so quickly.'

I can assure him that if he does this he will eventually be able to think calmly even of fear itself – without frightening himself.

If I could only give all of you the courage to put my teaching into practice, not to try to find cure in new drugs, but to be prepared to take what comes, without tensely steeling yourselves against it, then I would indeed be leading you to recovery.

There is still so much to say. I know that some of you – the mother of six, for example – are so weary, so sensitized, you need practical help, not just words alone. You need some sedation and rest for a little while, perhaps a tonic, before trying to practise my teaching.

If you feel like this, why not discuss your situation with an understanding doctor, pointing out to him that as soon as you feel better, you have a positive plan of recovery? Unfortunately, some healthy young doctors do not understand how desperately weary some of you are – how could they? But if they see you are determinedly armed with a blueprint for recovery, their interest will be aroused and I am sure they will help you to improve your physical health.

So:

- ✎ Recovery lies in reducing nervous symptoms to normal intensity, normal frequency; not in trying to abolish them entirely.
- ✎ No one can completely banish *normal* reactions, and nervous reactions are no more than normal reactions exaggerated.
- ✎ Try not to make memory part of the day's burden.
- ✎ One night's sleep will not work a miracle.
- ✎ Try to accept yourself as you find yourself in the morning.
- ✎ Point the body willingly.

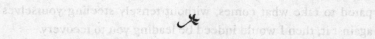

CHAPTER 10

Journal 2

Plan for Recovery

Tranquillization

Special Fears

Some of you who are afraid to travel from home, either alone or with others, have come to a standstill after your first successful efforts. So, I begin this journal with a talk on the kind of setback you may be now experiencing.

It is an advantage for a nervously ill person to work away from home, and I know from your letters many of you who go out to work are now not only moving more freely than you have for a long time, but are also less anxious when at work. There remain the many hundreds of sufferers whose work is at home – work that does not automatically provide opportunity to practise my teaching. They must make their own opportunities and these are the people who may now be needing special direction and help.

When they first used my book and records, and later the journal, they may have started off with enthusiasm and hope, and may have accomplished feats not attempted for years – such as walking to the end of the street, then as far as the shops, perhaps later entering a shop and even standing in a queue. When they did this, they may have thought they had conquered the world; at least, had a feeling of making progress, of getting somewhere at last. Now they are faced with the thought, 'Where do I go from there? What do I do next?' It is as if they have come to a dead stop, and begin to wonder if they have achieved anything at all.

These people are at a standstill because what they can do now – at least, without too much difficulty – has become so much part of their everyday life, the doing no longer seems an event. More important still, at the back of their mind lurks the thought that to be really cured, they must move further afield. They know recovery now lies along the rougher roads and they baulk at the thought. They stay hemmed in by their short walks, their small endeavours, and they feel they need a gigantic thrust from somewhere to make them take off along that distant, threatening, but beckoning way. At the same time, they dread anyone giving them that thrust. They both desire and dread simultaneously – an unsettling feeling, enough to keep tension alive.

PLAN FOR RECOVERY

The person who works away from home is rarely alone. He is with people during the day, even when travelling to work, and is usually with the family in the evening. The diversion that company brings relieves introspection and helps keep troubles in proportion. The person who need not leave home daily soon has to face the fact that she (it is usually a woman) must rely on herself to plan her own programme of recovery – one which takes her out of the house. She will also find that while the small goals are near at hand, reaching the bigger ones may mean taking journeys that seem not only impossible but – and this is important – pointless. There is little inspiration in taking a bus to such and such a place and then simply taking another bus home. To go in cold blood? Just there and back? That is asking a lot, especially on cold, dull days, when home fires seem so cosy. This aimlessness of their road to recovery may make such people feel even more aware of their illness as something unusual and hopeless – especially hopeless after having tasted the joy those early successes brought. This is why so many get stuck at this point. But remember, if like this, bogged down though you may seem, you have begun to recover. Any early success is a beginning and once made can never be quite lost or forgotten, however far down the ladder you may think you have slipped.

If there is a family cheering from the sidelines, the adventurer can at least announce later in the day that she went to such and such a place, or did such and such a thing. But even these lucky people have to go through the deflated feeling of returning to an empty house immediately after their big endeavour and must wait until evening to break the good news. This is difficult enough, but how much more difficult is it for the person with an uninterested family, or with no family. I would like such people reading this journal to take special encouragement.

I recently had the following conversation with a woman, which highlights some of the points just made.

PATIENT: I have improved my walking down the street by about twenty yards, but that seems to be my limit. Last week, there was one day when I couldn't even do that, so I went as far as I could and then came back and waited half an hour, and went out again in the opposite direction. I actually entered a shop and bought something. Now I can do that quite easily, so I think 'Where do I go from there?'

DOCTOR: Yes. These efforts begin to seem purposeless.

PATIENT: And yet it seems just as hard as ever to go beyond the boundary I set for myself!

DOCTOR: What is your next boundary beyond that one?

PATIENT: The town centre. I'm trying to walk there because I will be surrounded by shops. It is only another hundred yards further but I can't seem to make it. I can't get beyond the first twenty yards.

DOCTOR: You are making the mistake of trying to cope with the *distance*, of trying to get as far as the town centre. You all make the same mistake, you fix your eyes on a distant point and try to urge yourself towards it, thinking 'I *must* get there. I *must* make it!' Do not do it that way. *It is yourself you have to cope with*, not a certain distance or a special place. It is coping with yourself that matters, not 'making' the town centre. It is coping with *that one moment, the moment of extreme panic* – wherever you might be – that is important. When you go through any journey, whether it is only a few yards from home, or on towards the town centre (or even staying at home alone), I want you to understand that the worst you have to go through is *that one moment*. Even when you are in the town centre, surrounded by shops and people, surrounded by the *worst* that can frighten you, it is still *only the same moment* you have to go through. It is never very different. Never forget that! So please try not to be deterred by any threatening future event that may seem especially frightening. The very worst experience can bring you only that same moment. *Learn how to cope with it and you will have coped with everything.* I have explained how to cope with the moment of panic again and again in my book and records.

PATIENT: Yes, you have, and I know I did cope with it going up the street for those twenty yards; but going into town seems different.

DOCTOR: This is because you put a set objective, and strain towards it. Do not strain towards anything. Go moment by moment if necessary, and say to yourself 'I'm practising going towards the town centre. If I don't get there, it doesn't matter. What matters is that I learn how to cope with the feelings that arise within me as I go along.' How *far* you go is not important; how you go is the important thing.

PATIENT: But the further I go, the more panics I'll have to cope with and it is so exhausting, and if I get a long way from home, the panics will be awful and I'll still have to get back home!

DOCTOR: Getting back home will not be so difficult. A homing pigeon has nothing on you.

PATIENT: You are right. But what about all the panics that come as I get further and further away from home?

DOCTOR: You cope with each exactly as you coped with the one before it, by going towards it and not shrinking from it. You use the same recipe for each. Go slowly, wait and let the panic flash and spend itself. Sometimes it may seem to never quite die down, and may smoulder on all the time you are out. You can still function with this inner smouldering. Do not be bluffed by this. It is only sensitized nerves *recovering* from the blasts you have just given them, and quivering under the little blasts you continue to give them. I know you think you lose control of yourself during a real 'scorcher' and believe you cannot think. You can think, all right! You can think very clearly 'This is the end! This is it! Now I know I'm going to die! I'll have to get home quickly!' When you flash in this way, I want you to think just two words – utter acceptance. By utter acceptance, I mean let your body go as loose as you can, pass through the flash, and then go on with what you are doing. If you are driving a car, you may have to pull over to the side for a while before you go on, but then *go on*.

PATIENT: I'm not likely to be driving a car! But I know what you mean.

DOCTOR: I hope you do, because when you do it this way, you eventually reach a stage where you feel you could go on for miles. When you come through the worst and understand how you did it, the long journey unfolds before you as something you can cope with – because it can bring you nothing you have not already been through successfully. It no longer seems like a brick wall against which you are trying to hurl yourself. *The long journey unfolds*.

PATIENT: Oh dear! I know what you say is right. But can I do it? That's the point!

DOCTOR: Your body functions the same as the body of any other person; so why shouldn't you be able to? Treat it as I have advised and it must respond as any other body would. There is no special set of physiological rules for you. I am not asking you to rely on me, but on the fundamental laws of physiology.

PATIENT: What is physiology?

DOCTOR: It is the study of how a body functions. There is no such think as Dr Weekes' method. I teach nature's method. I am showing you what nature will do if you give her a chance.

PATIENT: I don't like nature one little bit!

DOCTOR: Of course you don't, the way you misuse her. I have a suggestion to make. Start off *towards* the town centre this morning, and don't turn back until you have tried to go through at least one 'blaster' with utter acceptance.

PATIENT: I'll try.

DOCTOR: Do not be disappointed if you fail the first time. The important thing is that you are willing to try. If you fail, wait where you are, and try again. Don't turn quickly and run home.

PATIENT: I think if I had a chance to stay out long enough, I could go right through this and then I would be able to carry on and get some feeling of achievement, which I find so hard to get now. I would be able to measure what I had done. I know I have made improvement, Doctor, but I am still only aware of my limitations. So many of us rush and we are back too quickly to an empty house and feel let down and frustrated because it seems such a little thing to have done, and we still have the day to get through. We can't keep trying because it makes us so tired. Speaking of tiredness, I do feel terribly tired. I am going out to dinner tonight, I have accepted that I am going, and I *am* going, but I feel *so* tired. Before, when I forced myself, I didn't seem to get so tired. Why is this?

DOCTOR: With acceptance comes a certain 'letting go'. One can nurse a sick patient for weeks without feeling particularly tired while the need is there; but when the danger is over, we may 'go to pieces'. Acceptance is rather like that. It means a 'giving in', and with giving in comes a slackening. This is excellent for desensitization, but until your body recovers its tone whatever relaxation you have achieved may seem like extra weariness. In time this passes.

This woman will now practise going towards the town centre. What of those who have no town centre so conveniently placed within walking distance? If you are like this, you must draw up a plan of action to suit your own locality. Plan two days ahead and then a day's break. Do not wait until Monday to begin; this will give you too much time to work yourself 'into a state'. Start this afternoon, if possible; also include part of each weekend in your practice. If after two days' effort and one day's rest, you feel especially tired, give yourself a longer rest. In the beginning when you first go out practising, you so often naturally do it the wrong way from habit, you become resensitized and are more easily fatigued. Hence, you may need extra tranquillization at this stage. I discuss this later in this journal. Do not wait too long wondering whether you are refreshed enough to practise once more. It is surprising how success refreshes and how failure tires. So do not wait too long in failure. Use your common sense.

Walk As Far As The Nearest Bus-Stop

Your plan should start with something a little more difficult than you have already tried. For example, if you have not been in a bus on your own, I suggest your first effort should be to walk as far as the nearest bus-stop. If the stop is too close, walk to the stop further on. If too far, walk half the distance. At least walk in the direction of the stop.

If you manage to reach the bus-stop, time your walk so that you will arrive there when a bus is due. If you can do only this much until you receive the next journal, it will have been a good deal to have done. Once you have made your plan, stick to it. It is easy to postpone it if it is raining, or you tell yourself you do not feel up to it. If you put off going, make sure you have a good reason.

Because I have asked you to walk only as far as the bus-stop, do not think I am discouraging you from boarding the bus. If it comes while you are there, and you feel prompted to take it, do so. Go to the next group of shops. Have in mind that one day you might suddenly find yourself in a bus, so plan now how far you would go. This will save some confusion on that great occasion. Do not feel compelled to board a bus at this stage. It is enough to practise walking to the bus-stop coping the right way with those moments of panic, those 'jelly-legs' and that faint feeling.

'I Would Almost Rather Panic And Get It Over!'

When you have truly learnt how to cope with panic, your fear of it gradually grows less, and as fear goes, so do 'jelly-legs' and faint feelings. This may bring its own strangeness. One woman said, 'When I do things now without the usual panic, it all seems so quiet; awfully peculiar. It is as if there is some kind of silent monster waiting to pounce. I would almost rather panic and get it over. At least I would feel alive!'

Recovery can be strange. The newness of successfully doing the ordinary everyday things that previously frightened you may make you feel unreal; you become apprehensive of recovery. Accept even this and realise that others besides you feel this same strangeness.

Make The Most Of Any Respite

You need repeated practice at accepting, until you have truly learnt your lesson. Your inner core or certainty comes only from repeated doing, and in the beginning 'repeated doing' at fairly frequent intervals, as suggested earlier in this journal. Do not let too many days lapse between efforts, but do not force yourself.

If you have been trying very hard and suddenly feel tired, flat and dispirited, wait a few days – even a few weeks, if necessary – until your spirits revive. It is so difficult to distinguish between real fatigue and only thinking you are tired, isn't it? Difficult to know when you should go on and when you should ease up.

The important thing is that once you decide to rest you do not fret because you are 'doing nothing about it' for the moment. Make the most of any respite.

The Little Things Remind You Of Other Occasions

When you have been practising the right way, even if much time elapses between practices, you will find that, while the contemplation of doing may still make action seem as difficult as ever, once you start moving the memory of your previous successes will help you. For example, if you have already made successful bus journeys and have temporarily reverted to dreading making another, you will find that once you are in a bus all the little things that go with being in a bus remind you of the other occasions when you managed successfully and your inner core of confidence will gradually come to life again, even if shakily at first.

No success, however small, is ever completely lost while you recover the way I teach you. It is the hard way, yes, but this is why you make your success part of yourself. You earn it. Setbacks may come, but even these will gradually pass, if you originally worked your way through your illness by your own effort. After the first shock of setback, courage will return. This may take some time, because you are indeed shocked by it; shocked to think it could happen to you, just when you thought you were so well; shocked at meeting so many of the old symptoms you hoped you had lost forever. *Let the first shock pass.*

I mentioned courage. Recovery is not built on knowing you had the courage to board the bus and sit through hell with clenched teeth. This wearies and discourages. Recovery lies in learning to sit in the bus with the right attitude. It lies in sitting there with utter acceptance of anything your body may seem to do to you, and more important, of anything you may think and so do to yourself.

TRANQUILLIZATION

I am assuming your doctor is regulating any tranquillization you are having. I make one suggestion: if you contemplate some big effort – such as a social gathering, a long journey – and find you build up much tension the night before (or the days before) extra sedation at this time is helpful; but first discuss this with your doctor. In time, with repeated 'doing', you will anticipate less acutely and extra sedation will not be necessary. Also it may be a good idea to discuss with your doctor the advisability of having a little added tranquillization during your early efforts to recover; when sensitization is likely to increase a little. I do not mean you should take additional tablets continuously, but only on those days when you are especially sensitized. Also, any extra dose should not be enough to make you lethargic. You need your doctor's help with this problem. He knows the dosage you are now on; he also knows you, and whether you are likely to become dependent on the extra amount.

SPECIAL FEARS

Since writing to you I have received over a thousand requests for journals. The fears you have confided in me when asking for the journals are the same fears my own patients have so often described. They are the fears most people have at some time or other, although perhaps not as acutely as you now have them. Which of us has not felt at least some of these: fear of being alone; of loneliness; of feeling inadequate; of ill health; of dying; of going insane; of fainting; of thunderstorms; of some animal – spiders, cats and so on; of not recovering from illness; of harming others while 'like this'; fear of 'ending it all'? None of these fears is so special. As I said, most of us feel some of them at some time –we take them as a matter of course. We took them upon ourselves when we chose to be human and not just animals lying in the sun. They are part of our existence and their nature does not necessarily make them part of a neurosis. They are very human fears.

The nervously ill, sensitized person is at a disadvantage because he feels his fears so acutely that they are magnified. Sometimes when he is particularly tense, agitated, a special fear may strike mind and heart so suddenly and with such compelling force it feels as if he is assailed by a power outside himself.

Fears That Spoil Life

People who are not nervously ill are able to keep their fears in perspective; their reactions are not severe, so that they can place the fears beside the joys of ordinary living, and in this way the fears play only a small part in their life. The nervously ill person's fears may be so strong they do spoil his life and may be so constantly with him that they can mar any so-called happy occasion.

Once again, as with the symptoms of stress, it is the intensity not the nature of fear that usually matters; to recover, one must reduce one's fears to normal intensity. One cannot hope to be rid entirely of all fears. I have yet to meet the person who has no special fear in the background, but it is *kept* in the background, kept in proportion.

Reducing The Intensity Of Fear

There are several ways of reducing the intensity of fear. Firstly, as mentioned in Chapter 5, by discussing it with a wise counsellor (doctor, religious adviser, friend) who may help the sufferer to see his fears from a reasonable point of view. He may need many discussions at frequent intervals before he can see reason and draw comfort from it. This is where a doctor's tape recording of an interview with a patient is especially helpful; he can play it many times daily, if need be. *It is possible eventually to adjust oneself to special fears and live happily in spite of them.*

Secondly, after discussion and being given a new approach to understanding a particular fear, the sufferer must be prepared, for the time being, to continue to react acutely when he thinks of his fear. He must learn to pass through each fear-flash and go on quietly with whatever he might be doing, at the same time practising seeing his fear from the new approach his counsellor (or maybe these journals) has given him. With practice, the fear gradually lessens, so that eventually he keeps a continuity of interest in his work, even as fear strikes. When fear no longer hinders, it gradually loses importance.

Desensitization to a special fear takes time and patience. I call this approach 'glimpsing'. Glimpsing works, but it is not easy and one must persevere for success.

It is comforting for a sufferer to know that many people share his fears and that they have managed to keep them within bearable limits. If they can, why not he?

What Causes Fear?

One could argue that some special fear makes a person ill, and that one has only to find the cause of the fear and remove it and the sufferer will recover. That sounds logical, and it often succeeds. Others say – remove one fear and the sufferer will soon find another to take its place: some may be even using their fears as an escape from facing reality. There is so much speculation when discussing nervous illness. Each doctor can speak with authority only from his experience with his own patients, and in my practice, to the best of my understanding, I have found that while some patients recover when the cause of the special fear is removed, many had originally been sensitized (as I have explained in my earlier book and records) by shock, accident, operation, difficult confinement, domestic upsets, and so on. While in this sensitized state, one or more of their dormant fears – the ordinary human fears we have been talking about – suddenly brought such exaggerated reaction, it became alive with importance and leapt straight into the centre of the stage. Also, any new fear that a sensitized person may feel may acquire magnified significance. Indeed, because of his sensitization, he now finds fear in corners where before he found none. This is sometimes called 'free floating anxiety'.

To put it another way, isn't it natural that if a sensitized person were able to dispel one fear, his sensitization would soon exaggerate another of his dormant fears? A sensitized person does not necessarily seek these fears for himself. They are already there. *His newly acquired sensitization vitalizes and magnifies them into importance.* I find my patients only too anxious to be rid of their fears and get on with their lives. Of course, there are always the old chronic work-dodgers, but I am not concerned with them here. I am concerned with people who are willing to try to recover. You are the kind of people who are willing to try to recover. You are the kind of people I am accustomed to treating – the people I have grown to respect, *whatever your fears, setbacks, failures*. I wish you all the courage to have another try. So:

- ℘ Recovery can seem strange. Accept even this.
- ℘ Make the most of every respite.
- ℘ No success, however small, is completely lost.
- ℘ Let the first shock pass.
- ℘ Recovery lies in establishing the right attitude.
- ℘ Relax to each fear-flash; let it pass and at the same time practise glimpsing your fear from the right point of view.

CHAPTER 11

Journal 3

At the Bus-stop

Right Reaction-readiness

Confidence

Going on Holiday

'At the bus-stop' can be translated into: at the station; driving a car; riding in the Underground; taking a lift; sitting through a meeting; indeed, making any effort which is especially difficult for a nervously ill person.

Some of you have succeeded in walking as far as the bus-stop; others have actually travelled by bus. Some have even made train journeys alone. Others have returned to work for the first time in years. These efforts are excellent; however, I hope you will understand that I am still concerned with those who have not yet found the courage to board a vehicle, or face any other dreaded situation, whatever it may be.

RIGHT REACTION-READINESS

Therefore, I now suggest a special exercise in our programme of recovery. I call it right reaction-readiness and you can practise it at home. Right reaction-readiness will help you not only to begin moving, or face any other special difficulty, it will also shorten the time of recovery itself.

By right reaction-readiness I mean one has prepared oneself to meet stressful situations the right way so often that the right approach is established as a habit; in other words, *the right reaction is ready*.

Those of you who still find achievement difficult do so partly because you remember so clearly your past failures and how you felt then; so, as soon as you think of going through such experiences again, your reactions are automatically those of dislike, panic, withdrawal. Unwittingly you are in a state of wrong reaction-readiness. Indeed, as far as wrong reaction-readiness is concerned you are in the front line of performers.

I hasten to explain that by right reaction-readiness I do not mean being tensely on guard to react the right way. Do not become caught in that net. I simply mean that one gradually establishes the habit of reacting the right way, both by mental preparation (the treatment I will now describe) and by actual performance.

We learn to play tennis by practising the correct strokes again and again, until finally we do them without thinking much about them. When preparing a concerto, a performer will practise slowly and pay great attention to detail and technique, and the more he practises in this way, the more groundwork he will have to depend on when he is actually on the platform waiting for the conductor to raise the baton. The more ground he has prepared, the more easily he will be able to rise above making the effort of physical performance to give free, inspiring interpretation. But the physical preparation must have been made thoroughly before he can forget the effort. By diligent practice he has laid down the necessary association pathways to bring him automatically the right reaction. Are you beginning to understand what I mean by right reaction-readiness? Let me illustrate this again by recording part of a conversation I had with a patient. He said, 'When I mentioned being on guard some weeks ago, I know now I was on guard to stop myself "listening in" and bringing on a "turn". I should have been on guard ready to relax and accept anything which might come. It's not like that now. I've learned to see a turn through, without reaching for the pill bottle. I can even work with the panic there. I'm not saying I don't mind it – I do – it's still horrible, but it doesn't throw me the way it did. I've learnt what you mean by "letting go".' At last he had the right reaction – relaxation with acceptance – and most important, he had it ready.

This brings us to the crux of the matter – how to make right reaction-readiness a habit. You can practise the following plan, just as you would practise anything else.

The Imaginary Bus Approaches

Sit in a comfortable chair and imagine you are in one of the situations – any demanding situation – you fear most; for example, if agoraphobic, that you are about to take your first bus-ride alone. While sitting in your chair, relax to the best of your ability, and then imagine yourself in this situation. Let us suppose you are at the bus-stop waiting for the bus. As the imaginary bus approaches, try to feel the same misgivings and fears you would feel if you were really there. Try to make your reactions as real and as severe as you can. As you experience them, remain as relaxed as possible and think, 'What would Dr Weekes advise me to do now?' Try to remember advice and practise *feeling* yourself following it.

Of course, I would want you to let the fears come, and be prepared to meet the bus *with the fear there*; to wobble on jellylegs if necessary, but to still direct them towards the bus; to let the panic come and not be deterred by any weakness that may follow. In other words, to accept the whole 'box and dice' and *move forward* with acceptance.

Reacting Freely

You may be so tired of hearing the word 'accept' that I will use another expression and say move forward prepared to 'react freely'. By that I mean to give free rein to all feelings – do not try to put a brake on any of them – let them all come. Do not fear that by doing this the feelings will be so overpowering they will immobilize you. The 'freely' saves you, cures you eventually, because it releases enough tension to encourage action.

It is possible that the term 'reacting freely' (or free reaction') may help some of you more than the word 'acceptance'. Different words, different phrases, have different effects on different people and 'reacting freely' is a good term. It describes well what I mean.

So, I would like you to sit in your chair and visualize the scene of boarding the bus, at the same time having the courage to try to feel yourself reacting freely. Having mounted the bus, find a seat at the front (not near the door in this bus!); even imagine yourself squeezing past the conductress and hearing her pass some disparaging remark about 'Can't you watch where you put your feet, ma'am?' Which, of course, is just what you can't do.

When in your seat remind yourself you cannot leave the bus in a hurry. Go through any emergency you can conjure up – even to the bus breaking down and your having to change buses – and as you feel fear, try to remember what I would advise you to do. Say it aloud and try to *feel* this right reaction. *The key to this practice is to remain as relaxed as possible while you imagine each situation you fear.* The more you practise, even if only in imagination, the more readily the right reaction will come when you find yourself actually in the situation. Indeed, after practising like this, you will sooner or later find yourself in a bus or train, or driving your car, or facing up to any other situation you have previously avoided. Do not be afraid to fail after practising this, but if you do, search for the reason, admit it and try again.

Behaviourism

Some of you may think the practice I have suggested is behaviourism. Right reaction-readiness differs from behaviourism in at least one fundamental. Behaviourism, with or without the help of drugs, aims at removing the fear associated with certain thoughts and experiences. Right reaction-readiness trains you by taking you through fear, not by avoiding it or trying to switch it off. The patient treated by behaviourism who has not learned how to pass through fear may find fear lurking in the shadows ready to come forward in the future perhaps in some new guise. There is only one way to reduce fear to bearable intensity without drugs, and that is by learning how to cope with it at its worst, not by trying to avoid it.

Fear-Removing Drugs

This is also my answer to those who have written for my advice on taking certain recently publicized 'fear-removing drugs'. Drugs have a limited time of action, so one must either continue taking them, hoping they do not lose their effect and have no harmful side-effects, or one must sooner or later wean oneself from them. When weaning time comes imagination can flash doubt in a second. The person trying to do without the drugs has only to think, 'What if I can't manage without them!' to panic and perhaps undo months of progress previously made with the help of medication.

The Only Way Out Of Fear Is Through It

There is only one way out of our fears and that is through them. Fear must eventually hold no fear, and it can do this only when we know how to quench its fire by losing fear of the fire itself. Free-reaction will, with practice, lead to right reaction-readiness and the two together will eventually lead to recovery. Start practising now, at home in your chair.

'I Can't Freewheel Quickly Enough!'

One woman wrote, 'I can't remember your advice quickly enough to freewheel past panic and other nervous feelings.'

The practice I have just recommended will surely help her, but I would rather she were not so anxious to 'freewheel past' panic. This is too much like trying to switch panic off. Because of such intense, well established wrong reaction-readiness, this woman asks of herself a physiological impossibility at the moment.

314   *Essential Help for Your Nerves*

This is why I have persistently advised you to find the courage to react freely and take what comes rather than try to avoid it – freewheel past it. Panic will cease to come of its own accord only when it, and other nervous feelings, switch themselves off because their coming is no longer significant. This will happen only when you have learned to ride through them so often the right way that deep within yourself you know that, even if they come, they will no longer overwhelm you. When true avoidance comes automatically in this way, from practice and more practice – and not only in your armchair – you will not have to struggle desperately to remember my advice, so you can 'freewheel' past your feelings; the feelings will dissipate themselves.

So remember:

✻ Practise free-reaction.
✻ The only way out of fear is through it.

CONFIDENCE

One man wrote, 'If I could feel confidence in myself, I would soon recover. I have very little social life because I am afraid of meeting people. Many of the symptoms described in Chapter 4 of your book *Self Help for Your Nerves* have left me, or come only on occasions. My chief concern now is loss of confidence. Other people seem so much more confident than I am.'

First, do not confuse what you think is confidence in others with what could be called self-assertiveness. So many apparently self-confident people are only self-assertive and they are vulnerable because of this delusion. They have never been put to the test, certainly not to the kind of test you are now meeting. Give them a crisis to meet and they may find their self-assertiveness of little help. There is no better way to develop real confidence than to come through experiences such as yours. You know how it *feels* to be without confidence, to *feel* almost a nothingness deep within you, so you are at least one step ahead of the self-assertive person, who has not had this valuable experience of self-knowledge. At least you are aware of this deficiency in yourself. I do not expect you to appreciate that this is already an achievement, but it is. You are not deluding yourself.

I know little about the man who wrote this letter, except that his work brings him into close contact with others who, because of his lack of confidence, I assume show their self-assertiveness in his presence more obviously than they realize, so that coping with them and his work may be a daily battle. He may force himself to meet these people on their own ground and then, after each trying encounter, sink back into himself to face a tiring, even trembling, reaction – natural enough in the circumstances, but interpreted by him as further proof of his lack of confidence. Also, this reaction may whittle away any small feeling of success he may have gained from having exerted himself.

For the moment, this man must be prepared to feel a reaction after any such trying experience, but he should try to understand it is a normal reaction to considerable effort; however, to effort which will gradually grow less when he is ready to accept the way he feels while making it, or after having made it. Confidence must come from within oneself and the price one pays is doing the difficult thing again and again. Successfully accomplishing the difficult once may mean only that at a particular time one had a special spurt of courage. Doing it often means the courage is no longer momentary, but has become inbuilt as part of oneself. One *knows* because of *repeated* doing.

No one need add up his failures. Each can be set aside. As I said earlier, *failure is not finality*. It is only as permanent as one allows. Failure has no will of its own. It hasn't a leg to stand on, unless we lend it ours. If you see failure only as a trial that did not succeed that particular time, but which may succeed the next time, then failure is no longer failure; it becomes an experience from which much can be learned.

When he finally learns how to face and talk to people by not being too impressed by his feelings of the moment, the writer of that letter will find it will no longer be important whether he *seems* confident or not. Now, he not only wants to *feel* confident, he dearly wants to *appear* confident before others. A truly confident person does not care whether or not he appears confident; does not mind admitting mistakes; does not mind being helped; does not mind asking questions – if they are pertinent. When I finally no longer minded looking up a long forgotten prescription in front of a patient, I knew I had arrived.

Tissue Layers

It is as if confidence is laid down in very thin layers – tissue layers – of feeling, day by day, month by month, each layer coming from the experience gained by making some effort, until at last the layers build up into established, deep, inner feeling. There is no experience more effective in providing those thin layers than the experience you are now passing through. Be glad of this opportunity to acquire real confidence, so you need not settle for self-assertiveness, as so many unfortunately do.

The last part of this man's report shows he is finding the right approach. He says: 'If I truly accept myself as I am, I will recover.' He will, and what is more, he will find that as he accepts himself more willingly, others will accept him more naturally. People will be more at ease with him. The effort will have finally gone.

So remember:

✤ What you think is confidence in others may be only self-assertiveness.

✤ Be prepared to feel a reaction after any trying experience. Do not give it undue importance.

✤ The price of confidence is doing the difficult thing again and again.

✤ One *knows* because of repeated doing.

✤ Failure is not finality. It has no legs to stand on, unless we give it ours.

✤ No experience can bring confidence more effectively than recovery from nervous illness, *when it has been coped with the right way*.

GOING ON HOLIDAY

How important it is to have an incentive to draw one out of the house. Spring is an incentive. This has been a dreary winter, following last year's disappointingly cold summer. As the warmer, brighter days now beckon you out of doors, you will begin to feel the benefit of my teaching. If you have a bicycle in the shed, prepare it for use. Some of you will think, 'How could I ride a bicycle while I am as giddy as this!' If you do it by concentrating on the riding and not on the giddiness, you will find that gradually the giddiness will ease. It is not so very difficult to ride with your type of nervous giddiness – the floaty, light-headed kind. Talk to your doctor, if you have not already done so, and get his reassurance that your giddiness is nervous. I can only assume it is. I have not examined you.

When you decide to ride – or walk, if you do not cycle – if possible, arrange to meet someone, or make a visit you have not made for a long time. Have the courage to be part of this spring. You can, by practising *free-reaction*. The key is in your hands. Use it. Do not be afraid to go out and hear the birds sing and feel the sun shine. It is all yours. Be part of it, at last. Look at the flowers; smell them; look at their colours. Enjoy them. All these things are yours. Go to meet them. Do not envy those who go out amongst them this summer; join them. You can, by quietly practising everything I have taught you. It works.

Shall I Go With The Family This Time?

And what of the holidays summer brings? Go. But go understanding that holidays can be disappointing for the person trying to recover from nervous illness. One can feel almost incarcerated in a small town or seaside resort, and if the weather is bad the impulse to rush home on the next train can be compelling. Many of you have had this experience and have returned home, dragging the family with you and deciding never, never to go on holiday again. Or if your husband has held you there against your will, what a miserable holiday it has been. You have counted the hours.

However, this time you take with you something you have not taken before – an understanding of what to do, a programme for taking a holiday. If you can see those first days through, you will find the strange, seemingly inhospitable place will not feel so strange. Indeed, you may find you do not want to leave it at the end of the holiday to return to the old familiar struggle.

A Mind Refreshed Is A Mind Unchained

To find no struggle at home, one would need to be away much longer than a few weeks – long enough for memory to dull the edge of the fears familiar surroundings can bring. Do not expect your holiday to do great things for you. Be satisfied if you have no more success than seeing the time through.

It could be that you gradually feel freer in those strange streets than you have felt for a long time, and you wonder how this could be while you feel so bound, so restricted, only one block from home. It is very natural. In a new place there are no upsetting memories and everything is an incentive. The streets near home are full of upsetting memories and no incentive. Change refreshes and a mind refreshed is a mind unchained.

On the other hand, the crowds, the laughter, the fun, may make you feel very aware of your 'strangeness', your difference from others. This too is natural. But remember, there may be many in that crowd going through a similar experience to yours. You do not look any different from them.

The Build-Up

When you decide to take the plunge and holiday this summer, the most difficult time will be the great anticipation, the build-up to going, and the first few days after arrival. See these two periods through and you will be heartened by the results. You may need extra sedation at night, even during the day, at that time. Your doctor should be consulted about this.

While you travel, do not think in terms of distance from home. You take your real home with you – your family and yourself. What you leave behind is a house, dear though it may be.

Do not let a house imprison you. Go forward as you travel and do not leave your mind behind.

Ride The First Shock

Don't be overawed by the thought, 'What if something terrible were to happen so far from home!' If you let this thought paralyse you into inactivity, you have already let something terrible happen and *at home*. One can cope away from home *by seeing all moments through without turning them into concrete barriers*. Whatever comes, *ride the first shock*. Take it slowly and the difficult moment will melt. This is the secret of losing the set-in-cement feeling and regaining flexibility of thought. When you can think more freely, you can move more freely. So go on your holiday this summer and treat it as another practice.

AGORAPHOBIA CAN BE CURED

It seems necessary to say definitely once more that agoraphobia can be cured. Please do not be impressed by anything you may read, or hear, to the contrary. When a person, whoever it may be, says agoraphobia is incurable, he is merely saying he does not know how to cure it. Doctors avoid 'claiming cures', but for your sake I am going to brush aside my natural disinclination to do so, and tell you positively that I have cured many people of agoraphobia. As an example, some time ago I spoke to a group of agoraphobic women in England. An Australian woman came to the meeting at my invitation. She came alone. When I first saw her, a year earlier in Australia, it was all she could do to make the journey to my surgery, even with her husband's help. She was cured enough to fly 13,000 miles to England, to move freely in

London on her own, even by Underground. She has now returned home and moves just as freely there. I assure you she is only one of hundreds.

Our Honorary Assistant Secretary has written this letter for your encouragement:

'I would not have thought a year ago that I would be writing a progress report. Such a thought would have been outside the realms of possibility. At that time, I was so deeply involved in the first major setback of my illness that to walk even a few paces from my front gate was enough to bring all the old terrifying symptoms. Failure piled upon failure.

'At no time did I lose faith in Dr Weekes's treatment, but I did lose the belief that I could make it work for me. However, with the support of the journals, I managed somehow to carry on practising, but in a very feeble way. I was frequently in such deep despair I felt what little effort I was making was too much, especially as I seemed to be getting nowhere. The prospect of giving up altogether was very tempting, although this too filled me with a feeling of hopelessness. This was where it became important for me to remember to "let time pass", if you see what I mean.

'After some months, I began to win small victories and was able to look back from one week to the last, and see I had progressed although there were still dark days; but after more time, even these became fewer. One day I was actually able to say I felt better and more at ease.

'At this stage, progress seemed to speed up (the word "speed" is purely relative here), although it was still some time before bad days just didn't happen any more. Now I feel relaxed and free to move around. I will not pretend I still haven't a long way to go, but I can view the prospect with optimism rather than dread. How glad I am I did not give up! To fellow sufferers I would say: "Never give up. Keep practising and letting time pass." I know some of you will think: "Oh yes, it is all right for her to talk but I just couldn't do it." But I know you can because I have come up from just those depths of suffering and despair you are now in, and courage is not one of my strong points. Believe me, from personal experience I can say, if you keep faith with the teaching in these journals, you will eventually win through.'

So remember:

✣ See the first days through, when contemplating going on holiday.
✣ A mind refreshed is a mind unchained.
✣ You take your real home with you.
✣ Do not leave your mind behind in a house.
✣ Ride the first shock. Go slowly and the difficult moment will pass.

CHAPTER 12

*

Journal 4

Floating

*

Flash-experiences

*

Low Tranquillization

Although much in these journals has been said about fear of moving away from home, the advice given can be used to help with other fears and problems. For example, the person concerned about feeling unreal has probably learned by now to understand this and not be too impressed by it. A feeling of unreality is a natural result of too much introspection and self-analysis, which brings withdrawal from outside interests. One should learn not to place too much importance on strange feelings in nervous illness. I stress this. A nervously ill person can be impressed so easily by unusual emotional reactions of the moment, because these can be made so intense and so flashing by sensitization. Flash-experiences in nervous illness are discussed later.

Even obsession – as I have repeatedly explained – is so often no more than loss of mental 'resilience' through extreme fatigue, and need not be a sign of a deep-seated neurotic tendency asserting itself, as some of my patients have been told. Often the nature of the obsession does not upset as much as the habit itself. Many obsessions are surprisingly unimportant in themselves, although they bring much suffering. Cure lies in accepting the presence of the obsession for the time being and in not trying desperately to get rid of it. Acceptance relieves tension and the fatigue that keeps the obsession 'engraved' on the tired mind. As one man put it, 'It is as if the top, thinking part of my brain won't work, and the lower, feeling part takes over.' He really hit the nail on the head.

I repeat: even those who believe their illness is much more complicated than agoraphobia can cure themselves by applying the advice given in these journals, which is based on those four principles – facing, accepting, floating and letting time pass. Of course understanding must stand beside acceptance.

I know this sounds simpler than it is in practice; but I assure you once again, it will not fail if you persevere with it.

FLOATING

I have often been asked: 'Just what do you mean by floating, Doctor?' so perhaps I should describe it more fully. Floating is the opposite to fighting. It means *to go with* the feelings, offering no tense resistance, just as you would, if floating on calm water, let your body go this way and that with the undulating waves. Let the moment of intense suffering float past you or through you. Do not arrest it, or stay baulked by it. Loosen towards it. Let your body go slack before it. Can you understand this? Some will think: 'How can I float past a whipping lash of panic?' You can, by waiting without resistance until the flash spends itself, and then by going on with the job in hand.

I speak here about letting the moment of suffering float past you, and again I sometimes speak of your floating through the moment. Floating can take many forms – you can imagine yourself floating forward through a moment of tense suffering, or you can imagine letting the suffering float through, and then away from you. They amount to the same thing – it is the 'letting go' implied by the words 'floating' and 'float' that matters. The important point is – floating is not fighting.

Although waiting without resistance may sound like doing nothing, it differs from apathetic doing nothing, because when practising floating you are prepared to go forward and face and accept. When you do this you are indeed doing a great deal. Apathy means no longer trying. One man wrote: 'Dr Weekes says, "Accept and let time pass", but I can't go on letting time pass. I've waited long enough doing nothing about it!' *I have never advised doing nothing about it*. You will never recover by gazing at the ceiling.

A young girl described her experience with floating. It may help you. She said on one occasion she was so tensed and agitated, when trying to enter a bank, she suddenly stood stock-still, locked in tension. She tried to push herself forward but this made her feel more rooted to the pavement than ever. Then she remembered 'floating'. She said, 'I stretched my arms out a little, and imagined I was floating through. It worked!'

What Is The Point Of Trying Again?

I have guided you through the past months, trying to gauge your progress – or lack of it – and trying to plan each journal to coincide with the stage of your illness. If you are progressing at the same rate as my patients in Australia – the usual rate – you are probably ready for a talk on setback. Although some of you have made train journeys, have driven your car alone, are doing your own shopping at last, you may now – because of physical illness, extra domestic tension, tension at work, or for no apparent reason – find yourselves in a setback which seems especially devastating after the early excitement of tasting a little freedom. You think, 'If I can do all that and yet slip back so far, what is the point of trying again? Why go on struggling, if it only leads to this?'

Nervous Illness Is A Lonely Business

Also, the family may begin to lose patience more than ever. The treatment sounds so simple to them. They may say, 'Why can't you do what the doctor says? She says just what we have been saying all along: "Take no notice of it! Forget it!" ' If only they could understand. Members of the family who have spent years being patient may suddenly find themselves so allergic to your illness they can hardly bear to hear it mentioned. And just when you need them so desperately to help you over these last disappointing hurdles. To you it seems so little to ask of them – that they stand by a while longer and not fail now when they are needed most. This may all add up to having recovery just within your grasp and then feeling it slip through your fingers for lack of extra help at a vital moment. Nervous illness can be a very lonely business.

Success comes to the one who goes on despite everything. You have not a hope of winning the race unless you are in it. Be assured that once you decide to stay beside the triers, even after a severe setback, you rarely have to retrace exactly the same painful steps when you begin to work at recovery again. The memory of past successes will come and strengthen your renewed effort.

So, do not keep comparing present poor performance with past success. Do not fall into the trap of thinking, 'Last week I could do that easily. Now look at me! I'm as bad as ever!' Do not allow last week's success to magnify this week's failure. Simply take each setback as an occasion for further practice.

COPE WITH YOURSELF, NOT A SITUATION

After a particularly successful month, one woman planned to make a journey she had previously found extremely difficult. It was driving alone through a long, lonely, narrow country lane. She wanted to see how she could manage now with her newly found confidence. I explained that her anxious wish to test herself could make her apprehensive and this, together with memory, could make that journey a disappointment. This is why I always stress learning how to cope with yourself and not how to cope with a particular situation. With repeated practice at coping with yourself until finally successful, one situation means little more than another. When you review your past efforts, whatever the situation, the efforts themselves have not varied so much, have they? Your field of endeavour is really a narrow one after all – no wider than coping with the feelings within you, feelings which, as explained in *Self Help for Your Nerves* and in cassettes, conform to a set pattern.

An especially difficult situation is no more than one which holds a greater number of difficult moments within yourself. These moments are not so very different in kind; they differ mostly in the degree of suffering, and are not necessarily related to the importance of a situation. Indeed, it is possible to have one's worst moment on what appears to be an unimportant occasion. When panic sweeps it sweeps, and when a sensitized person is going through a particularly bad spell there is very little variation in the intensity of the panic he feels. Try to remember this and let it help you not to be unduly afraid of any special occasion, or unduly impressed by a particularly severe wave of panic. This is why practising right reaction-readiness even at home, through teaching you to cope with yourself, can help you to cope with any situation.

PHYSICAL ILLNESS AND SETBACK

Many of the symptoms of physical ill health are the same as nervous symptoms; for example, palpitations, weakness, breathlessness, giddiness. The sufferer, after a bout of physical illness, has only to feel these mildly to be instantly reminded of all his other nervous symptoms. Memory works like a chain reaction. With fear and disappointment added, he may find himself in a setback, and this, together with the debility brought by the physical illness (possibly influenza), may make recovery seem remote.

You Do Not Heal Yourself

If allowed, time and nature will heal. Remember, you do not have to heal yourself. Nature is ready to do it, if you step out of her way and do not present her with those unnecessary obstacles, despair and disappointment. You remember to take your tranquillizers (how some of you remember!), why not take a dose of nature, three times a day? Say to yourself after each meal, 'Over to nature. I'll try not to hinder her by defeatist thinking.'

So remember:

- ✤ Go with the feelings.
- ✤ Wait without resistance. Let your body slacken.
- ✤ You will never recover gazing at the ceiling.
- ✤ Nervous illness can be a lonely business. However, you may not feel so lonely when you remember the many others tramping your way.
- ✤ Understanding now stands beside you.
- ✤ Learn to cope with yourself; not with a particular place.
- ✤ A special occasion is no more than another occasion for you to practise *coping with yourself*.

FLASH-EXPERIENCES IN NERVOUS ILLNESS

In my cassettes,* I said that if asked to pinpoint the most disturbing aspect of setback, I would say it is the return of panic when the sufferer thought he was cured. I would now like to add to this the recurrence of strange feelings which come occasionally, usually when least expected.

By strange feelings, I mean feelings that are difficult to describe; for example, a sudden feeling of dissolution; disintegration; of impending disaster; impending death; sudden flashes of

* For a full list of Dr Weekes' cassettes and recordings, and information on where to obtain them, see p. 425.

agitation; depression; apprehension; unreality; depersonalization. These feelings come at any time, perhaps even during an animated conversation, when the sufferer may be at his best, may even have forgotten his illness for the time being. Their effect can be so shocking he may suddenly be arrested in the middle of a sentence, a laugh. He may then think despairingly that he is able to go only so far towards recovery and will never completely recover.

The sufferer should learn to see these strange moments as no more than *flash-experiences* of no real significance. He must wait quietly for them to pass. *They will always pass*, and when not allowed to baulk him, will become no more significant than an occasional unhappy memory, such as we all have from time to time. Most people have collected a few strange thoughts over the years, which recur from habit and must be lived with. Life gives so much time to collect bizarre thoughts and feelings. When treated as unimportant, they are eventually hardly noticed. At least, they cause little disturbance.

It is a mistake to look for reasons for these flash-experiences. They should not be tracked down, analysed, and so unnecessarily accentuated. They are not worth it. Some, at least, occur to most sufferers during recovery and are a result of the suffering they have been through, and mean no more than that. Flash-experiences have no bearing on the future, so do not let them spoil a moment you may be enjoying. Be prepared to pass through the moment of shock or despair that they bring, without letting it distract you too much.

RECOVERY CANNOT BE HURRIED

The Honorary Assistant Secretary's letter has encouraged some of you to take great strides. However, I always have in mind those who still find the way difficult and who think progress, if any, is too slow. Try not to be upset by slow progress and above all do not be discouraged by your age. However old you are, you could not, in your present state, be spending your time a better way than by working towards recovery. So do not begrudge the time you give. Go quietly, at your own pace. No one can hasten recovery, not even for the sake of those he loves most. Hurry brings more tension. One can, of course, slow up recovery by not going forward enough, often enough. When I speak of hastening recovery, I mean feverishly trying to force the pace.

Never let setback put you out of the race. Toe the line again and practise the way I teach you. The teaching will not fail. Examine any failure and you will see that at a particular moment you did not have the courage to go forward. *You withdrew at the peak of suffering* and did not see it through. You shrank once more into yourself. No setback, however severe, can keep you from recovery if you are still willing to go on. Recovery always lies ahead in the doing.

LONELINESS

I wish to speak to those living alone, and this also means housewives who are alone all day, especially those whose husbands will not discuss their illness with them – indeed, in a few instances, will not discuss much with them.

A habit of fear is harder to lose in loneliness, because one's talking is mainly to oneself, and nervously ill people are especially poorly equipped to take their own advice. They have let themselves down too often in the past to be impressed by their own encouragement. Also, it is only too easy to repeat an upsetting habit when alone; there is so little diversion to discourage habit.

However, you are not quite as alone as you have been in the past. As I have mentioned earlier, understanding now stands beside you. Also, the knowledge that you are one of many people following the advice in these journals may bring a sense of fellowship.

By degrees this understanding helps relax your attitude even towards yourself – even towards loneliness – and as you become less interested in your own suffering, naturally you become more interested in outside events. In the long run, the best cure for loneliness is occupation among people, and each must find this in his, or her, own way. It is frustrating for all concerned that finding congenial work in good company should be as difficult as it is.

If you are trained for work, but have not had the courage to leave home to find it, pluck up that courage now and make the effort. Do not be put off if at first you fail at the job. You may have to go through many hours of misery before you accustom yourself to working again. Be willing to try; as I said before, you have no hope of winning the race unless you are in it. Fail as often as necessary, but no failure is as great as the failure to make the effort.

I wish each of you had some interest to help you face the day. Try to find interest. If you should think of taking a job, do not be put off by any journey involved; surely for a while someone would take you? If you have the courage to take the plunge and find work, do not be discouraged by any experience you may have during those first weeks. Those early weeks could not possibly be easy, anxious as you are. Go with the tide, 'tread water' until the worst is over. If you do this, the difficulties will iron out and you will find yourself gradually feeling secure in a routine which becomes familiar at last.

While at work, or at home, if practising my teaching, there may be times when you feel quite like your old self, only to find a little later that the moment has slipped away to leave you disappointed, weary. Wait. The happy experience will come again some other time. Do not try to force it, or hasten its return. If you do, you will only frighten it further away.

So:

* Never let setback put you out of the race.
* Try not to withdraw at the peak of suffering. This is the most important moment. Slacken; pass through.
* Go with the tide, tread water until the worst is over.

ACHIEVEMENT MUST BECOME ROUTINE

Recovery has its moments of spectacular achievement, but for any achievement to be established as recovery it must become routine. When this happens it may fail to impress you, and you may think you have made little progress. However, if you compare what you can do today with what you did a year ago, you will surely find you have made progress. There may be nothing spectacular, or even encouraging, about consolidating earlier successes, but so much depends on consolidation. Do not be afraid to give time to this, even it if means repeating often something you know you can now do well. Every little adds up and makes a firmer springboard to help you towards greater achievement.

One woman said recently, 'What is the use of trying to go there? I know I can do it now.' Knowing you can do it is not enough. If you rest too much on past achievement, you may find to your surprise that the next time you have to 'do it', you will have to break ground all over again. Repeated doing is always the answer.

The following letter came from the woman, mentioned in an earlier journal, who could not 'make' the town centre:

'Those who are still bogged down by the thought, "I can't do it!" may be interested to know how I managed to break through a little by deciding to really try to accept all that might come my way.

'I have been trying Dr Weekes's method since last September, starting by walking down the road a few yards. I did this daily unless I felt extremely bad – and gradually extended the distance. After a while, the short walks became easier and easier. However, instead of feeling elated, I felt dissatisfied. I was not satisfied with a small taste of freedom. I wanted complete freedom.

'My problem really started now, as I have not been able to bear my husband out of my sight for years. I went daily to his shop with him. This might sound wonderful to some lonely sufferers, but I assure you the dependency was crippling. I decided there was only one way to break it. I had to get a job. Of course, the mere thought of this brought back every symptom, but I had to choose between two evils. So I found work. I went for the interview, bearing the feelings as best as I was able, and started my part-time job.

'The first few days were terrible. I was separated from my husband; I had to take responsibility and was sometimes left in charge of the office, so that I couldn't walk out if I wanted to. I told no one of my illness. When I felt bad, I found taking a deep breath, and letting it out slowly, helped. I told myself it would all pass. And it did. My confidence grew until I could start off for work feeling only uncomfortable, but knowing I could cope.

'After nine weeks I had to leave the office as there was not enough work for two. I kept thinking they had found me inadequate and that I was not like other people. Along came setback.

My self-confidence sank so low, the thought of another job filled me with horror. I was also depressed by the waste of the effort I had so dearly made.

'I had discovered, by working like other people that most of the physical symptoms had left me, but depression and exhaustion remained. Yet I felt it was better to be depressed and exhausted when doing, than to have all the other symptoms that came when I was not doing. Now, locked at home once more, it was not long before I was flooded with the old feelings. Eventually, I realized I had to get another job. This time I went for the interview not caring whether I got it or not. This must have been a sort of acceptance, because I can honestly say I was not nervous and they took me on.

'I started working and to my amazement I did not feel too bad. My previous efforts were paying dividends. I have not been employed for three weeks. I still feel very tired, even slightly depressed, but I have a feeling this will pass. Through taking a *big* step I find I can do smaller things more easily. To act normally makes me feel normal. I have found the thought of doing is far worse than the actual doing. I am even at the stage where I almost welcome nervous feelings, so I can accept them and watch them pass. This is a step further towards coping with myself. Good luck to you all. Please try. It pays dividends.'

One man write: 'Since receiving your help, I have started work in a fairly responsible job but I cannot see myself completely cured. I frighten myself too much.'

At this stage this man should be reconciled to frightening himself for the time being. As I have said again and again, how can one expect to forget quickly fears that have upset one for so long. How could he quickly lose a habit of frightening himself while fear strikes at the slightest thought?

If he accepts frightening himself *as a habit to be expected at the moment*, and if he continues working with this habit, and does not immediately think that because of it he will not recover, his very acceptance will gradually desensitize him and in time he will be able to think about being frightened without necessarily immediately feeling afraid. This does not mean that, if he does this, he will never feel severe panic again. Of course he may. But if he applies the same principle each time and passes through the panic willingly, it will finally lose its power to dominate him as it does now. This takes time.

He is especially vulnerable at the moment in his new and more responsible job. He wants so much to hold it, he is probably constantly anxious about the way he feels. What more fertile soil could fear find! He should understand this also, and not expect too much from himself for the time being.

Second Fear Never Comes Unbidden

Some of you may think that sometimes you do not frighten yourselves, that panic comes unbidden and this is why recovery may seem so difficult for you. It is true that panic, as *first* fear, may seem to flash unbidden on occasions, but *second* fear (the fear you add yourself to *first* fear) never comes unbidden.

The above letter was obviously written in *second* fear. This is why I teach seeing panic through; teach learning to function with panic there, and not waiting anxiously to be free of it. Cure does not necessarily lie in being rid of panic. Cure lies in being willing to cope with panic when it comes and being willing to let it take its own time to go – because, believe me, it will take its own time. You can only hasten its going by not withdrawing from it.

Scuttling Back To Your Safety Zone

Real cure begins when panic does not send you scuttling back to your safety zone. The first time you discover panic no longer matters may seem so strange, you may feel frightened by the significance of your new discovery, and then, of course, panic can suddenly matter again. It seemed too good to be true. It takes time for sensitized reaction to the thought of panic to no longer bring panic. Time, time is still the answer, and willingness to pass through panic again and again, if necessary. But always remember 'willingness' (free reaction) is the key.

LOW TRANQUILLIZATION

A woman wrote, 'I am disturbed by the anxious feeling that comes when tranquillization is low.'

The anxious feeling that comes when tranquillization is low is really two feelings. One is the restlessness that sometimes accompanies the diminishing effect of the tranquillizer, and the other is the anxiety the sufferer feels when he realizes the effect of his tablet is due to come to an end. He knows when to expect this and waits anxiously for the time. As soon as he swallows another pill he feels better, even before it has had time to dissolve in his stomach.

Anxiety about low tranquillization may have as great an effect on one's body as low tranquillization itself. Here again, nature gradually compensates for the effect of low tranquillization, if the sufferer would give her a chance. *Remember, nature is always trying to adjust your body back to normal.* That is her constant task. The agitation that may come with low tranquillization must lessen if we hand the job over to nature and wait with acceptance. Agitation, although so disturbing, does no harm. It will always pass, *if you do not become agitated because you are agitated*. Beware of *second* fear to the best of your ability. One woman whose doctor withdrew her tranquillization wrote: 'I did have withdrawal symptoms in the beginning, which were unpleasant but only to be expected after four years of being on tablets. Because my body is no longer used to being constantly tranquillized, I now find half a tablet, taken occasionally, calms immediately.' Nature does do her work if you will let her.

I do not wish to minimize the effects of withdrawal of tranquillizers and am not asking you to stop your tablets. Some of you need them for the time being. In my opinion, if you take tranquillizers, the dosage should not be decreased until you have accustomed yourself to moving more easily. As you recover, you will find that from time to time you forget to take them. What a good sign this is.

Of course, some of you may be taking so may tablets during the day or night that the constant tiredness and possible depression you may be feeling could be caused by this medication itself, and not by 'nerves', as you now believe. Here it is essential to check with your doctor.

CHAPTER 13

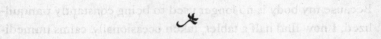

Journal 5

Special Encouragement

Home from Holiday

In past journals I have written mostly for those who have not been particularly successful. Now I draw attention to you who have done well, because recently depressing opinions have been expressed publicly about curing fears and phobias and I want to emphasize once more that fears and phobias – and this includes agoraphobia – are indeed curable.

SPECIAL ENCOURAGEMENT

Success must always depend on the treatment given as well as on the patient, and the essence of treatment is to teach the sufferer to go where he meets his fears, not only understanding them, but also knowing how to cope with fear itself.

AGORAPHOBIA IS DIFFERENT

Coping with specific fears – such as fear of animals, darkness, thunderstorms – is different from coping with fear of travelling alone from home. One can be taught to gradually look at, and think of, spiders, for instance, without fear, because this fear is of something *apart from oneself*. Agoraphobia is different. It is the fear of fear *within oneself*. If you are afraid of spiders, you fear the look, the feel, the bite, even the thought of the spider. If agoraphobic, you aren't afraid of the school hall, the restaurant, the train, the Underground, in the same way. You are not afraid of the actual places; you are afraid of the feeling of panic and the other sensations you have in these places. You are afraid of what is actually happening within yourself; afraid you will be unable to cope with it and of what this might lead to. Quite a different matter. I emphasize this point. So, if agoraphobia is given the same treatment as any other phobia, disappointing results are understandable. Agoraphobia requires a treatment of its own.

Courage Was Not Their Strong Point

According to reports, our Honorary Assistant Secretary's letter seems to have helped many of you because she said bravery was not one of her strong points. Many clung to this. They thought that if she could do it, then perhaps they too, who felt in their hearts bravery was not their strong point either, might have a chance.

To go out and face dreaded experiences does need courage. There is no question of this, but I am trying to show you that if you do it with the right attitude – with acceptance through understanding – by the laws of physiology themselves, you dull the edge of terror, if not immediately (though it can happen immediately), at least gradually. Actually, if you could realize it, you need less courage to face what comes when you truly accept, than when you go forward grimly under the tension of clenched determination.

The method I teach is a potent weapon in your defence because it is nature's way. Some of the reports in this journal show how readers who have not travelled for years can now travel freely at home and abroad by using this method.

Some nervously ill people are said to be of 'poor potential' and are accepted as 'chronics'. It can certainly be disheartening for a doctor to interview, for the first time, a patient accompanied by a thick pile of case-history sheets, including discouraging reports from other clinics. But the fact that the patient is actually sitting in the chair beside the doctor means he has a little hope left, and if the doctor can also find hope, good work can still be done. I have sometimes found that at the moment when I was tempted to think a certain man, or woman, would never make the grade, he, or she, showed the first glimmer of understanding and made the first step forward. It is essential that both patient and doctor stay hopeful. Hope is not merely a feeling. *It is also action – the first positive step towards recovery.*

While You Want To Recover, You Can

The wish to recover is the real potential. To put it another way: while you wish to recover, you can. So, however badly you may think you have failed so far, if you still want to be cured *you have the potential*. No matter what you think, no matter what the family thinks, what anyone might think, *you've got it*. You have it there. Of course, you recover more quickly if someone is helping you. And yet many of you are working from books, journals and cassettes alone. I wish I could give you personal help, but this is impossible. Your must manage by yourselves. You can.

Don't Wait Too Long For Confidence To Return

Some will say, 'I know what Dr Weekes means, but I just could not do it.' That is not good enough. There is no one who cannot do it. You can do it. Unfortunately, you have let failure disconcert and discourage you so much you now wait for confidence to come back of its own accord. Do not wait too long for confidence to return. It is regained only when you begin to do the things you think you cannot do. Even if the beginning is so small you can hardly recognize it as a beginning, it is still action, and *confidence is built on action*. You can sit at home and imagine yourself doing this or that, as I suggested in right reaction-readiness, but all the imagining in the world will not bring confidence *unless you follow imagination with action*.

It is not only the doing but also the knowledge of how you have done it that is important. The aim of some treatments today is to condition patients to act – especially travel – suppressing fear. But when conditioned in this way, are these patients acting with confidence? Suddenly a sight, sound, smell, anything which reminds, may start them panicking again. Do they know how to cope with panic? I doubt it.

This is why I teach you hard way – *by passing through panic to peace*. And it is because it is the hard way that some of you think you have failed so far. Don't blame yourself at this stage if you think you are among the failures. I am asking a lot from you, but the final reward is worth the effort. In the end you will have the confidence to cope with fear. But this takes time, so take fresh heart.

Some of your reports were especially pleasing. You admitted you still expected further setbacks, but were learning how to cope with them. People who have been led forward too gently by either having their emotions constantly calmed by drugs, or merely by suggestion, could find themselves very bewildered in a setback.

I want to qualify the statement 'by drugs'. From reports, some of you seem to think I am not in favour of tranquillization. This is not true. I said in the beginning that if you were severely sensitized, you might need enough tranquillization to take the edge off your too sensitized reactions, and here, of course, your doctor could help you.

He Need Not Go Without Some Tranquillization

In my practice I give tranquillizers as I judge necessary and reduce dosage gradually. One of the journal subscribers had changed his job for a more responsible one and said that although he was doing well he felt he needed help with some sedation during the day. He added he thought I would be disappointed about this. Not so; I do not expect him at this stage to do without such help. He may need help until he grows more used to the work. I know enough about panic to know it can cut through tranquillization, so he will still have opportunity to practise coping with it even while calmed a little by tablets. There is no point in enduring the added stress of a new job without some temporary help. Moderation in all things, even in one's attitude to tranquillizers. I make no hard and fast rule. In this matter, you must be guided by your doctor.

'I Don't Know How I Got Better'

A person who has recovered from nervous illness simply by time bringing him out of it – with no special treatment – usually says, 'I don't know how it happened. I just seemed to get better.' I am always a little anxious for such people because, should circumstances sensitize them once more, and should they become frightened, they can only hope they will come out of their fears as they did before. They often live in the shadow of apprehension. If you think my teaching is difficult, be cheered by the knowledge that this very difficulty, once coped with, will be your strength in the years to come.

To Find Someone Who Understands The Terror

In one report a woman wrote, 'I have been ill on and off since 1944, so I do not expect to recover in an instant. Looking back on last year, even I can see how much better I am. I can now take the car to go shopping alone. You cannot imagine how wonderful it has been to find someone who understands the terror and real hell one goes through. I didn't think it possible, and the fact that you know one's feelings so well has done as much to help me as anything. It is especially hard to make people realize how awful one feels when one is a buxom wench – and I've not lost weight; in fact, I've put it on, and apart from going a ghastly colour sometimes, I look fit to those who don't know me well.

'It is perhaps the feeling of utter exhaustion which I still find most trying, and I so often feel if I could only get my strength back I could cope much better with the business of recovery. I'm still frightened (petrified would be more correct) of going any distance from home – that is, to London or on holiday. However I feel by next year I shall be able to do these things, even if a little uncomfortably. I shall have a go. I still have giddiness and this is what started me off on the road to nerves. However, I am now able to cope with giddiness and loss of balance by floating and letting time pass. Now and again, I get flashes of confidence which are especially super.' Nervous exhaustion follows so much emotional suffering. It is sometimes the last symptom to go. It does pass.

So remember:

- ✴ Acceptance with understanding dulls the edge of terror. In the final count it takes even less effort, less courage to go forward with true acceptance than to go forward grimly.
- ✴ Hope is action, not merely a feeling.
- ✴ While you want to recover, you can.
- ✴ There is no one who cannot do it. You can do it.
- ✴ Confidence comes only when you begin to do the things you think you cannot do.
- ✴ Pass through panic to peace.

Sitting With Her Coat On

Another woman wrote, 'I can manage a short walk on my own and find that if I can do it on the spur of the moment, I am much better. It's the sitting and waiting with my coat on and trying to make up my mind that builds up the tension. As the evenings draw in, I'm going to try to go further afield in the dark. My biggest problem doing the short walks is the fear that people are looking at me, especially if I have to turn round quickly and come home. I convince myself that outwardly I look no different from anyone else, but the feelings still persist.

'I am able to get over the panic. Now, I just sit and wait. Recently a kind neighbour called and asked me to go to the shops with her. Although I've been going out only with my husband, I thought, "Here goes!" and I went and thoroughly enjoyed myself. I could not have done that six months ago.

'These may seem trivial things but, as you can imagine, they mean a great deal to me.'

Let me look at that letter and see how much more I can help that woman. Her trouble, of course, is mainly anticipation. When she anticipates, she should say to herself, 'If waiting is so bad, and I can manage it, surely I can manage going out?'

It is not only the nervous person who feels some apprehension when going on a journey. If one has been very happy staying with friends, or even has to leave home to go on holiday, the day of departure, even the day before departure, may bring a slight feeling of unpleasant apprehension. I call these the 'departure blues'. One who has had the habit of staying home for a long time would naturally feel this way to a strong degree if faced with moving far from home and to some extent when only contemplating moving a short distance away. Going anywhere out of the house becomes a real uprooting and this not *all* nervous illness.

Waiting Is The Most Trying Experience

So, if you have the chance of going out on the spur of the moment, do so. If you must wait before leaving, understand that waiting is one of the most trying experiences and that therefore you will possibly be agitated and upset. But be cheered by the thought that if you manage the waiting – as I have taught you – you will have gone a long way to managing the rest. You haven't gone out alone enough yet, you haven't succeeded enough yet, to be able to go out without some tense anticipation. *Time. More time. More doing.* This is the answer.

Anticipation is one of the last difficulties to go and doing things well one day and badly the next doesn't help anticipation one little bit!

Naturally, this woman has the feeling people will watch her when she turns back. If any of us, on setting off from home, remember something we have forgotten to bring with us – or a gas jet left burning – and turn suddenly round and walk back towards home, we feel a bit of a ninny. So much of what you think is illness is natural reaction in the circumstances. You turn such strong searchlights on your every action, every thought, you set a standard of behaviour for yourself the non-nervous person does not bother to even think about. So do not be upset if you 'feel funny' and think people notice. Seeing someone turn suddenly is not important to the passer-by. Try to make it unimportant to yourself. Turn again, Whittington, but this time in the right direction.

A man wrote on behalf of his wife, 'I read the book in bed to my wife at night. Within two months a remarkable change has come over her. Her attitude has altered. However, she is not completely free because she finds meeting people socially still very difficult.'

Mixing with other people is difficult for nervously ill people, not necessarily because they are shy by nature, but because usually, due to their illness, they are trying to do two different things at the same time. First, they try to listen to what other people are saying, so that they can give some kind of sensible answer, and yet at the same time they are listening intently to their own thoughts about how terrible it is to have such little confidence, to feel so confused, and be in such an upsetting situation.

This dual role makes them feel like two people – one struggling to carry on a conversation while the other stands by listening, undermining. A difficult task for anyone; a harrowing experience for the nervously ill person who needs so little to agitate and confuse him. Is it any wonder such a person avoids meeting people? However, it is essential for the woman mentioned in this letter (and for all like her) to understand that this strange experience must be lived through with acceptance many times before she will be more interested in the other person's conversation than in her own feelings and thoughts. In other words, until she can be natural.

Go Prepared to Feel Strange

I hope this explanation gives some of you the courage to go out and get the practice you need. Go prepared to feel strange; to follow little of the conversation; to feel awkward – even in another world; to make strange answers sometimes; but at the same time to know that while you feel this way so do many others and that to go through this experience is an expected part of recovery. How strange recovery can be, and yet not so strange when one realizes every phase is shared by someone else.

There is nothing odd about recovery, nothing unique about it, nothing really strange about it, except to you who experience it. What a well-trodden path it really is. There is no other way of getting used to meeting people, except first going through the difficult process of meeting them.

Repetition Can Establish The Pattern Of Your Illness

So much in nervous illness is weariness of doing the same thing, meeting the same people, repeating the same routine. Repetition can so easily impress upon you the pattern of your illness. One repeats the same performance almost as if under compulsion. Even the progress you have made, when repeated often enough, seems part of the old pattern. Going out, meeting new people, widens your horizon, gives you something new to talk about, and what is more important, new to think about. This refreshes; the old tracks of suffering are given some respite, so that when one returns to them, they do not sear quite so severely.

Remember, failure is part of recovery. I have not seen a patient recover without first failing somewhere, somehow. So, however you fail, you are still in the mainstream with many others. Recovery is still there, waiting for you.

There are many letters I would have liked to include here to cheer you. Here is one cheerful note. 'We have had a wonderful holiday this year and I have just moved house. I can now move freely and have no tranquillization. If I am a little apprehensive about a journey, I carry the journal or your book in my bag. If a spasm comes, I can carry on working and know it is not important and will pass.' Bravo.

Another woman wrote, 'More often than not, I can float through the frightening symptoms. It is easier now to toss them over my shoulder. The biggest problem, which has lasted many years, is tension and this makes muscles ache in a different place each day. Despite this, the difference and improvement is amazing. I'm sure I'll win through one day.' I'm sure she will.

A happy mother wrote, 'Today, October 1st, will go down in history for me. After twelve weeks of learning to drive, I took the car out of the garage myself this morning and picked up my young son from school for the first time. I was really jittery and said to myself, "Come on! You've got so far, don't give in!" And taking my courage in both hands, I did it. I have never taken drugs, so I have to rely on my own strength and the help in these articles. It's like conquering Everest, but I know now, it can be done.'

So remember:

⚹ Departure blues are natural. Reluctance to move far from home is not *all* nervous illness.

- When you have managed waiting, you have gone a long way to managing the rest.
- Tense anticipation is one of the last experiences to go.
- So much nervous illness is not more than natural reaction in the circumstances – but very much exaggerated.

HOME FROM HOLIDAY

After holidaying successfully away from home, you may dread returning to your restricted orbit. What you think of as your orbit is not so much barriers in locality beyond which you will not travel, as barriers in thought – mental blocks – beyond which you shrink from thinking. You are restricted by a habit of thought to the tracks you have followed for so long. So, when you return home, it is easy to fall into the old way of restricting movement within the familiar orbit. This is understandable, because at home so much reminds you of the old pattern, and so disarms you and weakens your resolve to extend your orbit.

Away, you moved in new tracks; saw new sights, different people; heard new sounds. These made new images in your mind. Playing golf on a new course, swimming, walking, meant a whole set of new pictures. You felt different, because you were different. You were emerging from the greyness of repetition.

As the day of leaving for home approaches, some of the old agitation could easily return. This is understandable. Don't immediately lose heart and think your holiday has done you no good; that you will never come out of your illness. It isn't easy to give up a new-found sense of freedom. It could be the first time you tasted freedom, after years of feeling caged, and it is not easy to stand by and watch it slip away.

Also you are disappointed because you sense that if this holiday could have lasted even a little longer, you could have consolidated the progress you made. As well as this, it isn't easy, having tasted freedom, to return to the place where the old restricted pattern of movement must be faced. It is almost as if the cage doors are waiting to shut behind you.

Take heart. After you pass through the first shock of returning, some of the newly found confidence will return. If the old suffering comes back when you reach home (and you may go looking for it before you even begin packing for home), do not immediately think, 'What's the good!' and doubt if you will recover. Most sufferers doubt. Recovery is such a new experience, you will surely misunderstand it, misinterpret it, because habit and memory are waiting to discourage you at every opportunity.

Into The Spin-Dryer

However deep into the spin-dryer of suffering you may go when you return, try to remember this gruelling experience will end, though for the moment you may seem to lose contact with everything that means recovery. However deep, however tragic the moment of setback may seem, try to glimpse that you are going through a temporary experience *which is still part of recovery*.

Have the courage to think, 'Even if I have to go through the ultimate in suffering all over again, let it come!' Have you ever really faced the ultimate? The fear that can hold you back from doing so is the fear that can keep you straddling two worlds – the world of nervous illness and the world of recovery. So, return with understanding and willingness to face whatever memories the old familiar scenes may bring and know that memory and its fears are also part of recovery.

Try to remember:

✤ You are restricted by a habit of thought.
✤ However deep into the spin-dryer you may go, the experience will pass.
✤ Invite the ultimate. When you do, the moment will melt.
✤ Setback and its fears are still part of recovery.

※

CHAPTER 14

Journal 6

Depression (Depletion)

※

Change of Life

Many of you have asked me to talk about depression. Although you may not realise it, you really mean will I talk about 'depletion', because the depression that comes to a person suffering from nervous disturbance is so often based on physical depletion following so much anxious suffering for so long.

DEPLETION

Depletion depends on depth of suffering, not merely on the length of time one has suffered. Vital resources are drained. There may still be a desire to do things and yet a feeling of inability to get stirring to do them; or there may be no desire to do anything. Sometimes desire may be fleeting – here one minute, gone the next – and all this makes ordinary living unendurable.

'He Could Get Better If He Really Wanted To!'

It has been said that many nervously ill people could get well if they really wanted to. Do not let this statement worry you. I assure you that while it may be true for a few, the vast majority want to recover; however, when a person is depleted, recovery may seem so beyond his reach, it may *appear* he does not wish to make the effort; even making an appointment a few days or weeks ahead may seem too much. To accept an invitation for lunch on Wednesday week is more like a threat than a promise of enjoyment. The desire to go comes only in flashes – if it comes at all – and Wednesday week, after days of dreaded anticipation bringing more tension and hence more depletion, can hardly be counted on to give even one flash of positive desire to go. So, on Tuesday night another ingenious excuse will be offered to cancel the appointment. What remorse, what bewilderment follow, what desperation of ever leading an ordinary life again. Had the friend said, 'Come today', the sufferer would have stood a chance of mastering courage and going, even if with inner turmoil. To plan ahead demands so much from a depleted person.

Packing a suitcase to go away is one of the most difficult tasks. It hardly matters how the case is packed, or how the lid is closed. If someone else will pack it – even one of the children – so much the better, and the packing may be started days before departure, so arduous the task. How odd it all seems. How unendurable. How difficult to explain. And what guilt it brings; what misunderstanding from some relatives and friends.

'Come On, Mother!'

Depletion is one of the most discouraging experiences in nervous illness. It is difficult to understand, difficult to cope with, and it calls for a lot of sympathy for those who feel this way. Unfortunately, it may have such an effect on the family; the joy of living can be dampened for them also, so they need sympathy themselves and may become incapable of giving it to the ill relative. Despairing families say, 'Doctor, what am I to say? Everything I do or say seems to be wrong.' A husband may say, 'My wife is beginning to build up such a hate session towards me. I can't understand it. She used to be so loving. Now she can be quite nasty and this is spoiling our relationship. What am I to do about this?'

This cycle can be stopped. Rarely has the family been coping the right way. How could they be expected to? – they are not doctors. They are likely to say, 'Come on, mum! Come and see Auntie Jess!' or, 'Come and have a game of cards with the Johnsons. It'll do you good!' Mother perhaps makes the effort, but often returns only temporarily helped, or more tired and dispirited than before she went. This is disappointing to the family, but especially disappointing for mother. Unfortunately curing nervous depletion may take some months, and trying to push or pull mother, or father, towards cure rarely helps.

The sufferer often calls depletion 'exhaustion', and it is close to exhaustion. I say 'close to', because however exhausted we may think ourselves (from whatever nervous cause), we are never quite exhausted. There would always be enough strength left to run downstairs if a fire started upstairs. Nevertheless, the depleted person often thinks himself completely exhausted.

If you suffer like this and can think of your body as temporarily depleted, rather than depressed, and understand that in time it can heal itself by recharging its emotional battery, hope comes into the picture.

The 'Horse's Hoof' On The Chest

Look at the people around you. Most of them have no more to help them enjoy life than you would have if you were well. Why then is it so difficult for you to enjoy yourself? It is difficult because your usual vital responses are weak. There is either a vacuum where feeling should be, or there may be a feeling of heavy pressing depression (the 'horse's hoof') on chest or abdomen, which may become so distressing that the cycle of depression goes on and on, bringing more exhaustion, more depletion and, so, more depression. There is nothing so depressing as depression.

Depletion can work in many strange ways. Anything which usually is only slightly offputting may seem exceptionally so; a depleted person may tremble before the slightest tense experience. Also, what previously had seemed no more than odd – for example, something as simple as a carved wooden figure – may appear disturbingly grotesque to a depleted person. While reaction to the unimportant – such as the wooden carving – can be exaggerated, one's reactions to more important situations seem weak or even absent.

When you understand depression as part of depletion (extreme fatigue) and accept it as a physical state, and are prepared to wait patiently (very difficult!) for your emotional battery to recharge itself, a time comes when you can talk to yourself encouragingly and *feel* the encouragement mean something at last. You can almost feel yourself lifting yourself up on to a higher level. You feel a little steadier, even though some of the sinking, exhausting feeling may still persist. For your own encouragement to mean something is indeed a step forward. In the depths of depression one feels one gets more help from others than from oneself, especially if they understand and offer encouragement. This is why one so often longs desperately for kind, helpful words from family or friends. Encouraging words seem as solid and supporting as a stout staff when said at the right time.

As The Lights Come Out, The Spirits Usually Lift

One of the perplexing aspects of depletion is its return from time to time when one thought one had completely recovered. For example, the old bogy may raise his head at only a slight disappointment, a mildly melancholic atmosphere, slight tension, and so on. One is reminded that reserves are still inadequate to cushion these experiences. Also, any one of us has moments when life seems less inviting than at others. Dusk is a low ebb for many, especially if the family which once returned at this time has now scattered. However, as the lights come out and the evening settles, spirits usually lift. So do not allow dusk to depress you unduly. Think of the thousands of others who share these moments with you, and maybe you will feel less lonely.

Some people are in such a state of depletion that they need complete rest, and this is when I recommend sedation – not heavy, but enough to keep the sufferer contented to do little for a week or two. The stage of severe agitated depletion does not last long if adequately treated and willingly accepted, especially if it is passed in surroundings which give some diversion or encouragement. Unfortunately, such surroundings are not always easy to find, despite the family's endeavours.

'I'd Like To See Myself Potter, With All This Work To Do!'

If adequately treated, the sufferer should be able to potter about by the end of a month. Those forced to continue at work may think, 'I'd like to see myself potter, with all this work to do!' But I am now talking only about a few extremely fatigued people. The majority of letters that come from those of you complaining of depression and exhaustion show that most of you can, and still do, manage to cope with the day's work. If you are like this, it helps to remember that this is a physical condition and it has arisen partly through trying to thrash a flat battery. If you do not want to make the effort to play cards with the Johnsons, do not make it, and do not feel guilty because you have not. But you must, at the same time, have an attitude of *moving towards recovery*. When I advise not making a certain effort, I do not mean you should make *no* effort. Use common sense. Waiting as optimistically as possible, without whipping yourself along, is more help than continuously trying to force a weary body. I use the word 'continuously' because unless you sometimes make effort you so quickly lose confidence is being able to do so. Please use common sense. I know it is not easy for a nervously ill person to decide what is the sensible thing to do. Then let me say, whatever course you take, *if you take it willingly and go with it*, you will be on the right track.

Nature's Gift

The vitality to bring interest even in the small happenings of every day is our legacy as human beings. It is there for each of us. Do not be misled by your temporarily depleted vitality into thinking ordinary living is not interesting. When we are well, even going to see if the plumber has done what we asked of him can be interesting and not just another chore. It is because you are as you are that ordinary living may seem humdrum, depressing. Remember this, and be prepared to take each day as it comes (especially the mornings) and say to yourself : 'My store of vitality is low because my body has been whipped by anxiety. I have overdrawn on my emotional reserves; even so, my body will heal itself again if I will allow it. This is nature's gift.'

It is not easy to say this and mean it, when one's mood changes so quickly: Hope, despair, hope, despair. Will they ever level out into ordinary living? They will. But as one recovers it is sometimes difficult to know how much 'not wanting to do' has become a lazy habit and how much is genuinely due to remaining depletion. Extreme depletion brings such definite symptoms, it is only too readily felt and recognized as a physical state. As depletion eases and depression lifts, one does the obviously interesting things easily enough, but still has the feeling of not enough interest to do the unpleasant things. There are many chores that most of us put off as long as we can – writing letters, menting, certain shopping, certain telephone calls, paying bills, and so on. Acute reluctance here is no more than normal reluctance exaggerated. Everything cannot suddenly be interesting. Everything is not interesting. So coming out of depletion and coping with the usual uninspiring jobs is always difficult, but must be done to reach a level where ordinary living becomes worth while.

Trust In The Miracle Restored Vitality Will Bring

So, try not to let the depression of depletion overwhelm you. Trust in the miracle restored vitality will bring. If, for instance, while you wait for recovery you find you can read only a little, that your concentration wanders, then read only a little. If you find it difficult to talk to people, hard to be interested in what they say, do not be upset by this. This too will pass and you are not always to blame. Some conversations can be very dull. Think in terms of depletion, not depression. This helps, because you can understand how a body can replete itself, whereas it may be difficult to understand the way out of depression.

There are some who pick at food constantly when depressed, but the truly depleted person's stomach often objects even to the thought of food. Depletion is a biochemical disturbance, so it is essential to take the right nourishment while trying to recover. Therefore, I suggest you discuss a tonic with your doctor — vitamins and, if necessary, iron. One should not take iron as a habit. Your doctor will tell you whether you need it. If you have only been picking at food you probably do.

A Low-Grade Gum Infection

Also, with depletion, one's mouth may have an objectionable taste, which lessens appetite. This may be due to a low-grade gum infection, or pockets of infection between teeth, and treatment with Vince dental powder can bring quick relief. Shake a little Vince into the palm of your hand and scrape it up on to a dry brush. After making sure the powder gets well between the teeth, spit out the excess saliva (the Vince forms a mild froth) but do not rinse your mouth. Let the Vince do its work for about ten minutes before washing it out. Use the Vince three times daily until your mouth feels normal; then once daily at your discretion.

A depleted person is sometimes deficient in calcium and this is best taken as milk. At least a pint of milk should be drunk daily. If you feel you cannot take too much solid food, do not forget the egg flip with sugar and a drop of flavouring essence.

She Seems Different Away From Home

Some people can be depressed at home and yet on going away can snap out of the depression quickly, only to find depression descending at the mere thought of returning home. When emotional reserves are low, mood can respond surprisingly quickly to environment. When away from home there is stimulation and spirits rise accordingly. It is almost as if this person is a mirror in which the environment reflects itself, so that he, or she, feels quite different while away – not even tired. Such a person needs a change in the home routine. Even a job for a few half days weekly can work wonders. The days at home are then grasped as opportunity to get necessary work done and are no longer a stretch of boredom to be somehow lived through. If the sufferer is a woman, brightening up the kitchen helps. So much time is spent there.

Also, working away from home, if it can be managed (I have not forgotten I am speaking to some for whom leaving home is difficult), opens new tracts of thought, even if it is only disapproval of the office girl's new hairstyle. If you are agoraphobic make the effort somehow to bring a little change into your life. At least think in terms of remediable depletion and not of depression.

So:

❧ Think of yourself as temporarily depleted rather than depressed.

❧ Your emotional battery will gradually recharge itself if you give it the chance.

- Wait as optimistically as you can manage.
- Everything cannot suddenly seem interesting.
- Trust in the miracle restored vitality will bring.

CHANGE OF LIFE (MENOPAUSE)

So much has been written about the menopause, it may seem unnecessary for me to mention it here. However, many women have asked if, and how, it can affect a nervously ill person, when trying to recover the way I teach them. I can answer this question simply. The menopause may have no noticeable effect, or it may make emotional reaction (already exaggerated by sensitization) more easily aroused. You will notice I have not said it will make the reaction more exaggerated. 'More easily aroused' is the crux of the matter. One point I wish to stress: hot flushes are not the prerogative of the menopause. They may come to any of us at any time, especially in hot weather. So do not think a hot flush or two heralds the 'change'.

Old wives have hair-raising tales to tell of the 'change of life', but when pinned down to facts, one often finds they themselves did not have such a bad time; they merely knew a woman who did. Most busy women pass through the menopause with little disturbance. One doctor told me it was the only time in winter she could go to bed comfortably without a hot-water bottle. Even so, too frequent hot flushes can disturb even a busy person. One's doctor can break the cycle of hot flushes with hormone tablets. These should be taken as a restricted course and gradually diminished. Taking too many courses is not wise as it only delays the menopause and may start uterine bleeding which can be a nuisance; one can never be sure if the bleeding is caused by the tablets or by something else, so the unlucky sufferer may have to go through several tests unnecessarily, before the innocence of the bleeding is established. While ovaries gradually stop functioning (and this is the basis of the menopause) other glands adjust the hormone balance. Taking too much artificial ovarian hormone interferes with adjustment. Acceptance is once more the safest course. It would be, wouldn't it?

The more easily aroused emotional response can confuse a nervously ill person, whose emotions are easily enough aroused, goodness knows. Tears and exasperation are already too near the surface; panic flashes too easily. Also, this expensive use of emotion may flatten the emotional battery and the nervously ill person (or even the non-nervously ill) may, during the menopause, find herself easily depressed. Understanding why this happens and that it will pass does help.

Occasionally some women have a few flushes ten years after their true menopause. We call this the 'little menopause'. It passes quickly and has more curiosity value than importance.

Far too much is made of the menopause. It is a natural event to save bearing children at an age when to do so would be dangerous. The term 'change of life' should be abolished – if one knew how to abolish a term. This aspect of a woman's life simply changes to become more comfortable each month. One should, of course, at this time, keep an eye on the bathroom scales. This is the time when an extra stone can creep on insidiously, and weight needs watching. Also, do not be tempted to throw off a jacket, or the bedclothes, during a flush. Too many middle-aged chronic bronchitics owe their chronic illness to this habit. See the flush through and you will gradually cool down. Another 'see through'! How often this principle must be applied.

Salt and water retention three or four days before a menstrual period can physically and nervously disturb some women.

Tablets can be prescribed to eliminate excess fluid and warning given to avoid salty foods, and too many cups of tea (too much fluid), during the pre-menstrual days.

A LETTER FROM CANADA

'After receiving the fifth journal, I decided to write about my progress and my hang-up. My general practitioner is very happy with what I have done. I am pleased also. He saw me through twelve years of not being able to do anything, and he felt helpless as I could not follow his advice. I was too terrified to try. Then I bought your records, book and now journals. The records are my salvation. They gave me just that something to get me going, also the fact that you said I could do it. I've had pretty strong setbacks; at one point I though I was right back at my very worst. But I pulled out. However, I have a feeling of "What now?" as if, maybe, I'm cured; although I know I'm not, as you will see as you read on. I just don't get the elated feelings I used to when I did things; also no enthusiasm. Maybe I feel no challenge? I'm even working for the first time in twenty-two years. I rather think I am almost at a cured point. I could be feeling normal and not recognize it. After being anxious for twelve years, I believe I've forgotten what it is like to feel normal.

'I hope you can understand what I am trying to say, although I cannot quite put it into writing. For example, this is one of my frustrating hang-ups: after going through a week of hell anticipating a hockey game, *the* night came and I went without any of the fearful feelings I had had previously. Crowds bother me as a rule, but there were 13,000 people at that game and except for slight dizziness, I had no anxious feelings. I was happy, but I did not get that elated feeling I thought I should have had.

'I can do this and yet in a small coffee shop I still have an awful time. There are other small things left I cannot do. This is what is so puzzling. I don't seem able to handle a small coffee shop. I've been practising for three months, at least once a week. I try different shops in different areas, but always have a bad time of it. I have not tried having dinner out, as I was hoping to do this gradually, step by step, starting with the coffee shop. I've said, "Come and do your worst!" but I am still happy to get away. I've heard others express the same thing. I wonder if going all the way into a crowded restaurant would help at this point? I just do not know.'

You Can't Eat Your Cake And Have It Too

I am sure this letter illustrates the way many of you may now be feeling. Elation, the stimulator in the early stages, must go, as one gets used to doing things not done before. One cannot expect to continue feeling elated. How could elation possibly last? Satisfaction may continue to come, but such an acute emotion as elation is a rare visitor to any of us. No non-nervously ill person feels elated because he, or she, can sit through a hockey match; so when you no longer feel elated, you are coming up well to being like other people. You are beginning to take doing the difficult for granted. This is good. Of course it was wonderful feeling thrilled after so many years of suffering. But you cannot eat your cake and have it too! There may be odd moments of elation from time to time, when it may suddenly dawn on you this is actually *you* sitting amongst all these people, but unfortunately such a sudden realization is often followed by memory stirring the embers of your illness, and on comes panic again. That is only to be expected. So pass right through it.

You might ask: 'If this woman can manage the hockey game so well, why does she still have to suffer so much beforehand?'

The answer is simple. She is not certain she can manage well. She has not managed well often enough yet to dull the edge of anxious anticipation. More 'doing' is still the answer, even if without elation.

Also, waiting the week before the game reminds her so much of all the other outings anticipated in misery, it recalls misery; but once she is at the game, she is reminded of the other more recent occasions when the doing has been successful, and this carries her through the ordeal. When she was ill and seldom went out, anticipation always meant dread, tension, fear of almost certain failure, and this is why it continues to bring such a build-up. The sufferer knows every minute of it only too well. That week of dreaded anticipation was not a 'hang-up', it was normal in the circumstances. It will be some time before the woman can take a hockey game in her stride, without thinking anxiously about it beforehand.

Gently, Gently Touch A Nettle

Now, the second section of the letter: the coffee shop. This is a good example of 'Gently, gently touch a nettle and it stings you for your pain'. The writer has been making the old mistake of trying to cope with a special situation and not with herself. (Rather like the person who can drive anywhere, even fly to the Continent, and yet finds walking up her own street difficult.) She asks would it be better if she were to go to a crowded restaurant. In other words, by doing a big thing she dreads, would sitting in the smaller shop seem easier?

It may, but it may not. It would seem easier only if she were convinced it no longer meant any special effort. She would have to convince herself very successfully of this. But I think she would go to the coffee shop in such a state of: 'Will I be able to do it now?' that she would be in worse suspense than before. So much depends on attitude, and when one is susceptible to flashing emotion, the right attitude is hard to maintain – the old flash knows its way around every corner. In those little shops she has suffered so much, the memories are all there waiting for her. While she thinks in terms of a place to be coped with, she could always be afraid of a small shop – any small shop – however well she managed the Ritz or the Savoy. In a little coffee shop, this woman is still withdrawing from the feelings she dislikes so much. And she wonders why they should come there, when they did not come at the hockey game. She says: 'Come and do your worst!' but she does not really mean this. She means, 'Come quickly and do your worst and get it over, so I can get out of here. And when you do your worst, do not be too severe, please!'

That Moment Of Panic-Crisis

That is not good enough. She must regard a small coffee shop as a place in which she has an opportunity to face the ultimate (that moment of panic-crisis) until it no longer matters. It is still the moment, not the place. It does not matter where she has 'the moment'; *it is coping with herself at that moment that matters.*

The writer of this letter still has to learn the trick of going towards panic with utter acceptance until she passes to the other side of panic. A little shop now seems more frightening because she is more exposed to close scrutiny; is closer to those around her, more afraid of being noticed if she should 'make a fool' of herself. At a crowded game, even in a crowded restaurant, she might feel bewildered by the noise and so on, but at the same time she is less conspicuous amongst so many, and is therefore possibly less vulnerable to her fears (especially if she managed to get a seat near an exit). But she is afraid of the same old fears, not the coffee shop. Onward soldier, into the coffee shop, *but withdraw from nothing* and don't hope to get it over quickly. Also, go more often than once weekly. See it through, again and again, in as relaxed a way as you can manage. As you do this say to yourself, 'Less tension, less adrenalin and, some day less panic.' This is a physiological fact. Rely on it. Your body does, so why not you? I know your body gets the message in reverse, 'More tension, more adrenalin, more panic' and responds to this. Try giving it the opposite message, the right one. The same physiological rules will apply, but perhaps not obviously at first, because of sensitization. Understand this, and do not let the slowness of response bewilder you.

When You Accept The Ultimate, You 'Let Go'

You might say, 'Dr Weekes has given me two different kinds of advice. One, to let it come and do its worst and face the ultimate, until it no longer matters; and then the other, to relax and so reduce the adrenalin which will then reduce the panic. Which am I to do?' There is no real difference between these two statements. When you accept the ultimate, you automatically 'let go' in attitude and this brings the relaxation that lessens adrenalin and so eventually lessens panic. But you do not get relaxation unless you really 'let go'. You will never get it if you say, 'Come and do your worst' with clenched teeth. So, when this person goes into the coffee shop, she should go expecting the worst and be prepared to see it through as often as necessary, with utter acceptance, and not be tricked into hurrying out of the shop as soon as possible. Halt! Go slowly, see the panic through. Stay there, until you are on the other side of panic. *You can do it.* This is the hard way, but it is the only permanent cure. Because it is the hard way – as I mentioned in Journal 5 – it takes time. So, do not question the time of your recovery, or think you are failing if you have not made much progress so far. If recovery is unduly slow, re-examine your attitude. You will find the clue to your failure there.

CHAPTER 15

*

Journal 7

*

Touching the Stars

*

What is Reality?

*

Take Yourself by the Hand

As usual this journal is for those still trying to get well; especially those who consider themselves unsuccessful so far.

'Unsuccessful' is a misleading word and some of you are tempted to apply it to yourselves when in a setback. Indeed, you may be tempted to think of yourselves as utter failures at this time, and be thinking seriously of searching for some easier treatment. And yet, if you look back to the time before you read my book and journals, and compare yourself with the person you then were, I think you will find that you have not been entirely unsuccessful all the time.

TOUCHING THE STARS

As one reader put it, 'I touched the stars, but I can't do it again, and I can't believe I ever did it!' This woman had, after weeks of apprehension, holidayed successfully in Switzerland. She had even floated past the staggering realization that the Channel lay between her and home; only to find, on returning, the old fears flooded back all too quickly. And of course they seemed so much worse after tasting that wonderful freedom while away.

But stars, because they are stars, can be touched only rarely. To feel one can grasp and hold the stars, one must have frequent opportunity to practise doing so, and that rarely happens in an everyday programme. Opportunity to practise my teaching is there in your own town, village, suburb, but how humdrum it seems in comparison to the excitement, variety and beauty of that successful journey away from home.

Coming back to the familiar brings so many small shocks. Nothing is more spirit-crushing than hearing the washing machine grinding noisily away at the holiday wash, as if nothing unusual had happened. One can almost hear it say, 'Come out of that dream, madam, and listen to me. I'm the one you must live with now, not those mountains, those lovely breakfasts by the lake. Wake up! It's time to switch me to spin-dryer!'

The Holiday Balloon Bursts

It helps if one realizes that the non-nervously ill person may also go through a similar experience of seeing the holiday balloon burst. Ecstasy is only ecstasy because it is short-lived. So do not lament if you cannot believe you ever touched a star; cannot believe you really did accomplish some outstanding feat. And don't be surprised if, despite the experience, you may feel you

Essential Help for Your Nerves

have made no progress when you return; may even seem unable to cope with the simpler tasks you managed well before going away. You will never lose what you have gained, if you give yourself time to settle in and do not prolong the process by revolting against it. Don't let shock, surprise, disappointment, throw you completely off your stride. Once again, let the first shock pass, and you will slowly gather the harvest of success you planted when you touched the stars.

Reading about holidaying in Switzerland may be tantalizing to those who haven't yet 'made' the town centre; but so many did holiday abroad after years of being housebound and wrote lamenting about the difficulty of homecoming that I thought I should mention it.

WHAT IS REALITY?

The feelings of a nervously ill person are important to him most of the time. This does not mean he is necessarily selfish, egotistical. He is simply so bewildered by his illness that he feels unable to be interested in other people, even in his family. He would like to care. How a mother would like to *feel* love for her husband and children, but her detachment can be so great, she is convinced she does not love them any more.

Emotions can always be deceptive, and in nervous illness *the emotion of the moment* dominate other feelings. For example, a husband's failure to say the right thing at the right moment seems more important than the year of companionship. One woman said, 'I know I must love my husband deep down inside me, but I can feel only exasperation at his actions and criticism.' Unknowingly, this exasperation may be mixed with envy because the husband can do so casually what the wife finds so desperately hard to do. What is more, the doing is so easy for him, he cannot understand why it is not as easy for her.

The Surface Waves Make So Much More Fuss

In her report, a woman described the upsetting, even fearful, thoughts she had about her children. If only she knew how many mothers write about this she would not think herself the monster she now does. I mention this particular fear so often in my book *Self Help for Your Nerves*, I am surprised to be questioned again about it. I wonder if this woman has read the book, or listened to my cassettes; because she goes on to say, 'I am trying desperately to put the thoughts out of my mind.' *This is the very thing I advise against doing.* The more desperately she tries to force forgetfulness, the more imprinted the idea will become. This is a normal physiological process.

Once more I stress that so much nervous illness is simply normal physiological process exaggerated and one cannot therefore blot it out completely; one can only reduce it to normal intensity. She must let her thoughts come, as is their habit, but she must understand they are only thoughts and try not to be too impressed by them. They are like the surface waves, not the deep current, and it is the deep current that helps carry the ship along. Unfortunately, the surface waves make so much more fuss than the deep current, and therefore seem so much more important. These frightening thoughts bring no truthful message, however forceful, real, they may seem. They bring a message only of habit and fear, and these are not reality.

Reality is rarely the feeling of the moment. The feelings of the moment change readily with attitude, and reality is too deeply implanted to change readily with attitude; it survives the feelings of the moment, but how uncomfortable and convincingly real those momentary feelings can be to the nervously ill person. Don't be bluffed by frightening or negative feelings of the moment. Try to release them, let them go, float past them. They are not reality.

Some of you will not grasp the full meaning of what I write here, or have written in other journals, until you actually experience it. Then you will re-read with interest and understanding. You may be surprised to find how much of what I write has new meaning when you re-read it from time to time. Therefore, I risk repeating myself, and will stress once more certain advice that is especially helpful.

1. Setbacks are so often memory and habit working together. Very rarely can one recover without them. So do not think you have 'slipped right back' if you happen to have a setback. Use the same method you used to come out of your illness. The more often you apply it, the more readily it will work.

2. Be consoled: the more improvement you have made, the more frustrating a setback may seem, so do not let a particularly severe setback discourage you too much. A woman in San Francisco said jokingly, 'I must be recovering, Doctor, because I'm having my worst setback!' Two months later she was able to travel to Paris, for the first time in years.

3. Physical illness, especially that frequent visitor influenza, can so deplete one's resources that the old symptoms of nervous stress return, or threaten to return. Most of you know that apprehensive feeling, when the old dreaded sensations hover and you are afraid they will really arrive. Let them hover; do not try to push them away, or run away from them – at the same time watching over your shoulder to see if they have really gone!

I know how possible it may all seem on Monday, and yet how impossible on Tuesday. Strange, how all the possible Mondays may still fail to convince when one impossible Tuesday comes along. Try to be patient through impossible Tuesday – even through physical illness – and trust in nature to repair the damage – with a doctor's help if necessary.

4. Recovery may be so new and strange, it is as if you have lost something you must find again. This something is your illness. Do not be surprised if, when you are most successful, the strangeness of success makes you feel odd. Don't be surprised if this oddness reminds you so acutely of your illness that you are beguiled into thinking you are ill again. It is almost as if you cannot tolerate recovery.

   You will eventually feel at ease with success when enough of it robs it of its strangeness. So pass through every such experience, until it no longer surprises and upsets you.

5. Wanting everything one minute and nothing the next is one of the most tantalizing aspects of depletion. Also, you may think yourself capable of doing everything one minute and then incapable of doing anything the next. This too is usual. Is it any wonder that I keep advising acceptance and warning against trying to delve for reasons for this or that?

6. I know that feelings often depend on circumstances and that when these change, feelings automatically improve. But there is the other side to the coin and this is not appreciated as much as it should be. When feelings are less intense, circumstances seem less overwhelming. The proof of this lies in the effect tranquillizers may have. After tranquillization, the impossible may seem so much more possible. So try not to be too impressed even by circumstances. By going towards them willingly, you lessen tension and problems may not seem so insurmountable.

7. The way to recovery is the same for most of you. Blasters come when least expected. Pass through. Pass through. *Always pass through to the other side* and never run away. Running away is such a waste of time, because once you have started to recover by using the method I advise you will always turn back and tackle that obstacle again. Wait. Gather breath for a new advance. It may take time and many changes of mind, but eventually, you will do it. Some who have discarded my advice and have tried other methods have written saying that after a while they have found themselves back in square one with the journal. Indeed, many have said they carry the journal wherever they go; and this conjures up such a picture of tattered pages amongst lipstick, purse and tissues, and of shaking hands rejecting page after page while frantically searching for a special passage, that I include here a short article which can be conveniently carried* and which will be especially helpful when trying to travel away from home. It was originally made as a ten-minute LP recording.

Again there will be repetition, but for those who still need help, repetition is treatment. Goodness knows, through fear and habit some of you repeat often enough to yourselves the wrong advice. Repeating the right advice – hearing it again and again – is essential. Don't think, 'I know that' and pass it by. It is not enough to just 'know' it in your head. You must really feel it in your heart. Do you really feel it?

* This article was detachable from the journals. Naturally it is not meant to be torn out of this book.

TAKE YOURSELF BY THE HAND (FROM A TEN-MINUTE LP RECORDING)

If you are suffering from fear of leaving the safety of home, you probably had an experience in the past that upset you to an exaggerated degree and, as I have already explained, sensitized you. So many women say, 'It all started after the birth of my last baby.'

If like this, you are not really afraid of open spaces, even of the supermarket. You know perfectly well that if you go to the corner store the grocer won't shoot you, the houses won't topple on you. You know none of these will harm you. So what are you afraid of? You are afraid of the feelings that arise within you when in this situation, feelings that seem to overwhelm you so that you seem unable to think clearly while they are present. You do not trust yourself while you are like this and this is why you are afraid to go out alone.

I will now take you out with me, step by step, and as we go will explain exactly what happens, why it happens, and what to do about it. Are you ready? Good.

But look at you! Before we've opened the front door, you have tensed yourself like a violin string. You thought, 'Oh, my goodness! What's going to happen now!' If one plucks a taut string it responds by vibrating, whereas a slack string does not. By tensing your body, you made it an instrument on which your fears could play a very painful tune, and you did this before you even put one foot outside the door. *This is your first mistake.*

Instead of tensing your body in anticipation of what might happen, let it go, slacken it, release it. Slacken those strings. The worst that can happen out there, in the street, in those shops, is that you can let yourself become frightened. I understand how severe that fright can be; but if you release as much tension as possible and are prepared to accept what happens, are prepared to surrender yourself to it, it won't be quite so overwhelming. Surrender, accept. Slacken those strings. Take a slow breath; let it out gently. Have you the idea? (Have you really got the idea!) Good.

Here Comes Mrs X

We are off. But, oh, my goodness! here comes Mrs X from down the street! What are you going to do about her? You advance towards her with your heart in your mouth. You can feel your heart thumping in your throat, banging in your chest. But your neighbour's heart is also beating quickly, perhaps just as quickly as yours. She is intrigued because she hasn't seen you out alone for months. Then why should your heart's quick beating be so specially frightening? So particularly uncomfortable? Yours is so upsetting because your sensitized nerves are recording and amplifying each beat. Does it really matter if you feel your heart beating? It doesn't matter in the least. It certainly does not harm your heart. So don't be afraid to feel your heart pounding while you talk to Mrs X.

But she is settling in for a good old gossip. What if she were to continue for another ten minutes, *half an hour?* You tremble at the thought and think, 'I can't stand it. I'll make a fool of myself. She'll notice!'

But now I whisper, 'Take your hand off that screw. Let your body slacken. Loosen. Loosen. Take a deep breath; let it out slowly and surrender completely to listening to Mrs X. She'll eventually stop.'

You hear me. You hesitate and then release the tension just a little, and strangely enough, standing there does not seem quite so difficult. You even feel a little pleased with yourself. And so you should be, because you have discovered something very important. You've learned Mrs X is not upsetting you, as you thought; you were upsetting yourself. *It was your hand tightening that screw, not hers.*

Now we are off down the street again. You feel a little better. You made it! But now you must cross the main road, and just when you need your legs most they suddenly turn to jelly. Those old jelly-legs. Did I say suddenly? It did not happen quite as suddenly as you thought. As you approached the main road, you became frightened again and fear released that old enemy, adrenalin which gave you the jelly-legs. The effect will gradually pass if you do not stay frightened by it and so add more adrenalin. But you do not understand this and stand rooted to the pavement, sure your legs will never carry you across.

Jelly-Legs Will Still Get You There

But here again I whisper, 'Jelly-legs will still get you there, if you will let them. It is only a feeling; not a true muscular weakness. Don't be bluffed by jelly-legs. Don't add more adrenalin by being afraid of them. Let them wobble. They can carry you across the street whether they wobble or not. And don't think you must hold tensely on to yourself to keep yourself from collapsing. *It's the holding on that exhausts, not the letting go.* So let your legs wobble. It's only a feeling, not a true muscular weakness.'

You crossed the road. You made it. By now you are not quite as impressed by the tricks your body has been playing on you. When you realize this, you somehow feel charged with new strength. But wait! You have forgotten the shop! There may be half a dozen neighbours waiting to talk in there! You may even have to wait in a queue!

In a flash you turn all the screws at once and give yourself the full fear treatment. It is as if you have made no progress at all, and just when you thought you were beginning to get the right idea. And while you look at the shop in despair, your body seems to sway; the street to swirl; the buildings to topple. Everything goes blurred. You clutch at a post to steady yourself. How are we going to explain this one? This is a beauty!

It is explained very simply. Severe tension disturbs coordination between your muscles and the balancing apparatus, and this apparatus receives the wrong messages. So, the buildings seem to topple and you feel unsteady. Also fear dilates your pupils and vision therefore seems blurred. This is so frightening that you withdraw from it; let it overwhelm you. But it is only the same old tricks in disguise, the same old turn of the screw. And as usual you turned it yourself.

Let The Storm Pass

Wait! Let the storm pass. Let the effects of adrenalin pass. Even at the climax of your fears, surrender and accept. At the very moment when your feelings seem to engulf you, that is the moment above all when you must surrender and accept. No more Oh, my goodness; no more What ifs.

If you do this, you will find you will keep the grip on yourself you previously lost. If you go forward, however hesitatingly, with understanding of what is happening, ready to accept all the tricks your fears may play upon you, your reactions will gradually calm. And, as I have explained so often, you won't have to try walking as far as the corner store one week, into town the next, until you finally graduate to the supermarket. You will find peace in the middle of the town square, *because you take your cure with you, wherever you may be.*

Just as you read this advice, say it to yourself again and again when you are out, until you make it part of yourself. It will never fail you if you follow it, and follow it until you learn to take yourself by the hand, until you are your own guide, your own strength.

A LETTER FROM BIRMINGHAM

'All the fears and sudden panic you speak about have been mine for years, except that I have never given way to confining myself to the house. But as you point out in your bulletins, in spite of the help your book gave me I continued to be plagued by them, though I am now trying to accept rather than fight them.

'Last November, a friend agreed to go with me on a cruise to the Canary Islands. I had not thought anyone would want to go anywhere with me.

'From the time of booking, I seemed less physically well than usual –pains in my middle, diarrhoea, and I was obliged to go to my doctor. He gave me various remedies, but the main advice was to step up my tranquillizers a little until I got going. Even the day before we sailed, I felt I could not go and only a good talking to from my doctor, and fear of disappointing my friend, made me pack and go.

'So with Avomine against sea-sickness and three tranquillizers a day for about three days, I went. I was not seasick and not once did I panic. I found myself talking happily to many passengers, and actually played two piano solos in the ship's concert. I took your bulletins and read them in bed occasionally. Even if we did not get the sun we hoped for, I feel I have gained my old confidence in myself, which matters more than anything.

'I have no doubt that when I next plan a holiday, even if it is only in England, I shall struggle with the same fears and have the same uncomfortable physical aches and pains, but I hope after this experience that I shall not be such a coward again. I am grateful to my doctor for the patience he showed me, and to the journals for showing people like me you don't think us the fools we often think we are.'

AN INTERESTING REPORT FROM KENT

'Some of you may feel, as I did at one time, that maybe other people may benefit from Dr Weekes's teaching, but that you are too much of a coward to manage it. May I tell you of my experience and how I realized that, no matter how cowardly one is, it works?

'Just recently, I had the misfortune, or, as it happened in the end, the fortune, to be a police witness at a Quarter Session trial. When I was told one Friday that I would have to appear as a witness on the following Monday at court, I spent the whole weekend working myself up, until I was sure I could not go. When you consider that I cannot go out alone at all, I think you will realize the worries I had.

'The police were to call and collect my husband and me by car and the journey there and back was 39 miles. We were to be there at 10.30 a.m. As most of you know, waiting is for many of us one of the worst things.

'The jury was not sworn in until 12.45 p.m. Then the court adjourned for lunch. My husband had gone for a walk and I was left alone in this large building. Before I left home I slipped a copy of one of the journals into my handbag, just in case. By relaxing and following exactly in my mind what I had read so many times in the journals, I was able to go up to the gallery and find the cloakroom. When my husband returned I was back in the main hall having quite calmly combed my hair and generally titivated.

'We went up in the lift to the cafeteria and had lunch.

'At 2 p.m. I was taken to the witnesses' waiting room. Now, of course, without my husband. This was the real test. It was followed by forty minutes of gruelling questioning in court. I did not feel one ounce of fear.

'How could I, such a dreadful coward, have done this? It was just by remembering what Dr Weekes had said. I did not even take the journal from my handbag. After all that time waiting, plus the forty minutes questioning when I had to go it alone, I feel a new person. So if you are like me, a real coward, listen to the words written in each journal and take heart.

'It works, really it does. Try again.'

Once again, I assure you, if you are prepared to do your part, you can definitely be cured. I would not spend so much time and effort writing these journals if I did not know this. I look forward to a better understanding of agoraphobia, and of the anxiety state in general, by doctors in the future and consequently to improved treatment.

✽

CHAPTER 16

Journal 8

Understanding Setback

✽

The Importance of Habit

✽

Struggling the Wrong Way

✽

Letter from a Woman who Suffered for 28 Years

I first wish to talk yet again about coping with setback. So many doctors lose heart when trying to help their patients cope with setback. And yet, if doctor and patient can understand and bear with setback, recovery is the prize.

Some of you have had moments, even weeks, when you have felt – to quote one woman – you could 'tackle anything' and then have had a setback, which – to quote the same woman – 'makes everything ugly again'. She also adds, 'I still find myself shrinking from my thoughts; at the same time, I almost see things in their right proportion, only to slip back into the old habits once more. I'm having a setback at present after a fairly good period. I feel terribly disappointed, and yet I know I'll build up again slowly.

'For instance, today I had a few moments when I actually lost my fear of my main phobia. It was the best moment in that direction. One learns an awful lot from breakdown. I look forward to the time when I can see it all in the right light. The intelligent part of me knows it is quite ridiculous, but fear seems always to hold the upper hand.'

THE IMPORTANCE OF HABIT

I would like you to appreciate the importance of the word 'habit', because so much of your illness is bound up in that word. Fear of this, or that, is *your habit*. This is why you seem to have things sorted out, see them clearly without fear for a while and then lose that reasonable glimpse. It is not so much that fear alone comes back as that *the habit of fear reasserts itself*.

When you appreciate the full meaning of habit, you will understand why setbacks come and why your progress seems to include so much going backwards, so much slipping back into old habits – rather like climbing a greasy pole.

The Forbidden Handbag

A woman carries her handbag everywhere. Suppose she were told she must never carry one; that she must go empty-handed. Do you really believe she would immediately adapt herself to not carrying a handbag and feel comfortable when going out? For months she would feel lost and make the gesture of looking for it before leaving home; make the gesture many times in many different places to see if she had it with her. Even months after she had thought herself adjusted to being without her bag, she could suddenly find herself automatically groping for it.

Recovering from nervous illness is like this. Should you lose your fear for a while, the you-behind-you (you know the 'you' I mean) is so used to being afraid that, from habit, it will go looking for your fear to present it to you again. If you could then think, 'This is only the return of the lost handbag!' and go forward through the fear, you would once more come out into the clearing.

In my book *Self Help for Your Nerves* I talk about the curtain lifting and then descending again. Also, I say that if you can but glimpse for a few moments daily without fear, you will have made a beginning. With practice, you will glimpse more readily and hold the glimpse for longer and longer, until it is the final established point of view. Then you will be at peace.

Glimpsing is a frustrating, painful process, as this woman's letter shows, *but it is part of memory*. So, do not think of those persistent efforts of the you-behind-you as failure; try to see them as an inevitable part of getting well. You are still improving even when being presented with the forbidden handbag. Habit dies hard, but in time it does die, if you see it through its violent protestations.

STRUGGLING THE WRONG WAY

The following is a letter from a woman who kept herself ill by misunderstanding and mismangement. I analyse in detail the sentence in italics.

'I am trying to follow the advice in your book' – she had not had the journals – 'but *I can't get over the first hurdle*. My trouble came on after a lengthy illness, when I began to have panicky feelings when out of doors. You say in your book to relax and take deep breaths, etc.; but this is my main trouble, *I just can't take a deep breath. I gasp and gulp and feel myself suffocating; which brings on more fear.*

'You also say "let time pass", but I have been ill so long *I must get better soon.* Life is passing me by and I am getting nowhere. *I feel such a coward and such a failure.* I used to be able to make myself do things I was afraid of, *but now all my willpower is gone.*

'*If only I could get out again without fear,* I could get my old job back. Please, *how can I control these panic spasms when I try to go out?* If I was all right when I went out, there would be nothing to fear and I could go. But now, feeling the way I do, I sometimes daren't even go to the bottom of the street. If a gasping panic comes on, I have to be near home so that I can get back quickly. *I feel I am going to faint and have to run home.*'

When this woman says 'I can't get over the first hurdle' she is trying to say she can't rid herself of enough fear to begin practising my advice. She stresses this when she says, 'If I could go out without fear.' She will never go out without fear while she puts off going until she is without fear. She has waited in vain for years to be without fear. Waiting and watching so fearfully keeps her nerves always alerted to respond in an exaggerated way, so she feels ordinary fear as panic. And the ground is so well prepared for panic while it is feared so much. Her anxiety provides the adrenalin from which panic is made. When she says, 'If only I could get out again without fear' she is really saying, 'If only a magic wand would remove my fears!' This young woman is looking for a cure outside herself. She won't find it – not a lasting cure. She must be prepared to go out *the way she feels now* and not wait until she is unafraid.

Essential Help for Your Nerves

She must not go tensely, hoping fear will not come. Fear will certainly come, so she must be prepared to be afraid, but at the same time try to release as much tension as possible, if not in her body (this may seem impossible at this stage) at least in her attitude. Once again I stress, she must go towards fear, not shrink from it, and must be prepared to let it do its worst. Only when she had faced fear and managed to see it through in this way will she remove the underlying apprehension and tension which are creating the very fears she fears. A habit of fear can be broken only when it is faced with acceptance. Only then will moving away from home – or any other dreaded experience – cease to be such an ordeal.

Once again I stress the difference between true acceptance and just 'putting up with'. 'Putting up with' means advancing and yet retreating at the same time. It means an attitude of Hurry! Hurry! Get it over quickly!

When first attempting to face and accept fear, speed in taking those first steps only heightens tension. Faltering steps – and they are faltering steps, almost like a child's – should never be taken quickly. A moderate pace gives you time to remember and practise what I teach. It gives time to collect the right attitude to panic – time to see how much you are frightening yourself. Speed encourages adding *second* fear and achieves nothing except defeat, because speed means running away, although you may be actually heading in a forward direction. *You can defeat panic only by giving yourself time to work with it.*

So, when you attempt to meet any situation you fear, *start slowly* and continue at a moderate pace until the end; *go even more slowly when panic reaches its peak*. Hurrying is agitation and agitation in a sensitized person sets the scene for panic.

Acceptance means a certain resignation and resignation implies a certain peace. A hunted criminal who finally becomes resigned to his fate and gives himself up finds some peace and this is not unlike the feeling the nervously ill person feels when he finally decides to surrender to the worst fear can do – when he decides to accept and not fight.

'I just can't take a deep breath. I gasp and gulp and feel myself suffocating.' Who wouldn't, if they fought for breath the way she does? But she will not suffocate, because her lungs will expand enough despite her efforts to thwart them. She is thwarting them with her tense struggle. She need not worry about taking a deep breath. Shallow breathing will do, *if she pants with acceptance*. As the tension passes, her chest muscles relax and breathing becomes normal. Even if she gulps and gasps, she won't suffocate, because, as already explained in my first book, there is a breathing centre in her brain which automatically controls her breathing in spite of her heroic efforts. Surely she has gulped and gasped often enough without suffering to prove this to herself.

'I must get better soon.' Once more she is creating tension by putting a time limit on recovery. But how understandable this is. She has been ill so long, she is desperate. To be patient seems almost impossible. But impatience means more tension, more sensitization. She must try to be reconciled to giving as much time as necessary to recovery. In the circumstances, what better way could she spend her time than working for recovery. She must surrender even to this.

'I feel such a coward; and such a failure!' Why should she? She has struggled heroically for years. Few understand how much she has struggled and suffered. She has failed only because she hasn't known how to succeed, not because she has not tried. Every line of her letter shows how she struggles bravely, but the wrong way. Exhaustion and despair, not cowardice, have almost stopped her in her tracks.

'I used to be able to make myself do things I was afraid of, but now all my willpower is gone.' One can almost feel the lashing she must have given herself. 'My willpower is gone' is simply another way of saying, 'I have so exhausted myself with fighting and getting nowhere, hope has gone.' Who wouldn't be tired of tilting at such windmills! The majority of nervously ill people, including the most intelligent, seem naturally to take the wrong road and *fight* their illness. I hope by now you see the difference between fighting and accepting?

When one surrenders and accepts, the act of going out, or doing anything one is afraid of, may at first continue to be grim. Indeed, in the beginning it may seem especially difficult, because facing and accepting demands more energy than resting at home in defeat, and the nervous person usually has so little reserve, she thinks she simply hasn't the strength to try to recover this way. As she learns to accept this temporary additional tiredness, the keen edge of panic gradually dulls just a little, and she builds strength and hope on this 'little'.

'How can I control these panic spasms?' She can't immediately, because she is sensitized, and she can't turn panic off like a tap. One can't expect to control directly a whipping flash which, at times, seems to come like an electric shock. The control is *indirect*, and as I have explained so often, comes only by learning not to add panic to panic. Only in this way can she begin to desensitize herself, until panic gradually grows less intense.

'I feel I am going to faint and have to run home.' She feels she is going to faint, but she can still *run* home. If she can run back towards home without fainting, surely she could *walk* towards the shops instead? She is not running away from fainting. She is running away from the fear she will faint; *from the fear that makes her feel faint*. When headed towards home, her fear decreases, so naturally she feels less faint.

If she would practise walking forward in the way I have stressed so often in these journals – by letting her body do whatever it wants to – tremble if it must, feel weak if it must, *even faint if it feels like it* (this takes a lot of acceptance!), she would find, behind the trembling and the faintness, the strength to move forward , however hesitatingly. She would not faint.

Each despairing statement in this letter was based on a misunderstanding which entrenched her more deeply in her illness. Surely it is time for her to try a new approach, directly opposite to the one she has been using. Is not this the approach I teach?

LETTER FROM A WOMAN WHO SUFFERED FOR 28 YEARS

'I am at last beginning to make some progress. As I found the early stages of recovery bewildering and believe this is not unusual, I thought others, struggling as I, might be interested to read of my experience.

'When I first read Dr Weekes's book, I thought here at last was an explanation of how to cope with my illness, because the more I studied her method, the more it seemed right. I agreed wholeheartedly that curing the state I was in was the important thing, and not trying to find an original cause. I never could understand how finding a cause hidden beneath twenty-eight years of suffering could help me now, even though most of the psychiatrists who had tried unsuccessfully to help me had thought so. To take myself into my own hands, regardless of the past, and not look for outside cure to make recovery easy, was a challenge I knew I must face at last, if I was to recover.

'Did I have the courage; the staying power? Could I do it? Had I been ill too long? Could I stay convinced this was the right way to recover, even if others tried to convince me it was not? Did I have all this? Others had managed, so why shouldn't I?'

I Took Off With Enthusiasm

'My immediate reaction to the explanation of sensitization and how panic occurs was one of relief and hope. I decided to try the basic theory of facing, accepting, floating and letting time pass. I must say the thought of letting more time pass filled me with dismay, as half my life had gone in illness. However, I took off with some enthusiasm and achieved minor successes in making moves I had not made in years. "Can it really be as easy as this?" I asked myself. "Surely there must be more to recovery than taking off in a flash this way." I soon learnt that for me there was, because the early elation passed and I was back where I started.

'I know now the first elation merely masked my fears. The real start had to come more slowly and not so emotionally. I studied Dr Weekes's method until it became part of my thinking. So much so, that one day I spontaneously took off in a bus and travelled a short distance from home. This was the first bus I had boarded in twenty years. I was excited, but when I reached home I was so exhausted I could not believe I had been near a bus.'

Minor Successes Followed By Fatigue

'For weeks this cycle repeated itself – minor successes followed by fatigue, but no real feeling of growing confidence. Each adventure seemed too great an ordeal to bring lasting confidence. But I could not lose the glimpse of success I had had when first doing these things. I had touched something I was unable to grasp and hold, *but I had touched it.*

'I realized that while some could go out immediately and never look back after reading Dr Weekes's book and listening to her records, others would find the method hard. I had to accept that I was one of these. I remembered her words, "Each recovers in his, or her, own time. Accept even that." Realizing this method would work for me only if I were willing to accept it fully and let the cure come from inside myself, in its own time, I accepted the time involved at last.

'It was hard to think cure had to come from me, for I had always hoped for cure from an outside source. And yet, however hard I found doing this by myself, a little voice inside me kept niggling, making me stay the course.'

Supertension, To Be Met As Any Other Form Of Panic

'On one occasion, after I had managed to travel some distance from home, everything seemed to recede and I felt so completely lost I felt incapable of asking anyone to help me home or hail a taxi. this was different from flashing panic. However, remembering Dr Weekes's method, I managed to think, "Meet this the same way as panic. Wait. Take it slowly." Finally I was able to hail a taxi. I realized that what I had suffered was no more than supertension and had to be met the same way as any other form of panic.'

Progress Seemed A Dream

'Progress still seemed a dream, although I was learning so much. I managed successfully one day and failed the next; was sure one day, despaired the next. I became desperate when I heard of fellow sufferers, also using Dr Weekes's method, who were making quicker progress than I was. I suspected I might not have what it took to stay in the race.

'At times my illness seemed a safer way of life; at least I knew where I stood and it sometimes seemed better than being always on the emotional yo-yo, up one minute and down the next. But once started, I could not give up.'

This Was My Last Attempt

'A few days later, I drove round Hyde Park on my own. Panic after panic flashed. When I returned home, I was so spent and upset I nearly vomited. This, I decided, was my last attempt. I would stop the whole thing now. But somehow, I didn't feel the relief I expected. That wretched little voice kept niggling. Where had I gone wrong? Why had I failed?

'Trembling in every limb (because I suspected that wretched little voice would make me try to do the journey again), I analysed where I had made my mistakes. Suddenly, I knew I had accepted nothing. I had tried to get through the journey at the fastest possible speed and had withdrawn from panic by trying to blast my way through it. My one thought had been, "Get home at all costs!"'

I Set Off Again

'I decided to drive round the park again and this time try to make a success out of failure. I would try to learn from my mistakes.

'After a good dose of glucose, I set off again, very, very slowly, prepared to meet panic when it came and to try not to add *second* fear. On that first journey, I knew I had added so much *second* fear. At my special panic-spot, I slowed down almost to a crawl. Of course I panicked, but I saw the flash right through and kept going forward slowly, but willingly, with the car. I did not panic again. Don't ask me why, but I didn't. Three times I repeated this journey. I saw at last that recovery could begin to work only from actual experience and that that was why it must take time.

'I now became almost obsessional in my desire to experiment with myself. I was afraid to let a day pass without doing something new. I thought that if I did, I would lose the progress I had made. This was a mistake, because it led to more tiredness. I was trying too hard. I learnt to take even the aspect of recovery more sensibly. If I missed a day or two, I stopped whipping myself.'

In The Line of Fire

'In spite of feeling I am now on the right track, and in spite of feeling real hope, I am sometimes nervier than when I was in the shelter of my agoraphobia. This, Dr Weekes explains, is because I am meeting situations I have avoided for years and am putting myself in the line of fire for further panic. It is obvious that the road to recovery may temporarily bring increased sensitization and this makes us feel as if no progress has been made. However, if we repeat some of the earlier steps, we will find they are surprisingly easy. For example, the other day I found entering a big store alone effortless. This came as a surprise, because I had formerly done so at great cost. This gave me hope.'

My Illness Had Been My Reality

'Recovery sometimes makes me feel so unreal, I have to keep remembering Dr Weekes's words, "A feeling of unreality during recovery is normal in the circumstances." To me, for twenty years, my illness has been my reality, so I suppose it is only natural these new experiences should feel unreal. I do understand that only when "going it alone" is not a novelty will my changed way of life begin to feel real.

"Setback, exhaustion, depression, panic, all seem failure. Yet, I have learnt that I cannot go forward without them. This is a hard lesson to learn, because it is not easy to put oneself voluntarily into positions that may bring them.

'Although I am only at the beginning of this road, I have had those moments of glimpsing. They have brought me such hope that I feel to turn back now would be impossible and I fear going forward a little less.'

THE SAME WOMAN, EIGHT MONTHS LATER

'Since my last letter, I have had to come through a severe setback following an operation. All went well during the first part of January. Driving around Hyde Park and going into a store held no more fear. Even on a bad day, I could see the panic through and come out on the other side. To take a bus was an everyday occurrence. I had even driven through Richmond Park alone and had waited in a queue there. Also, there was a marked change in my attitude. I felt more positive as a person and was meeting domestic crises more calmly. This change was reflected in my work.'

Would The Glimpse Hold?

'Could this be what I had waited for during those twenty-eight years? Would this glimpse really hold? Could I go further? Dare I be sure? My feet were only touching firm ground and I knew it. Then suddenly, for the first time in my life, I was faced with an operation. It couldn't have come at a worse time. If only it had given me a little time to consolidate that glimpse. But things rarely work out that way. Indeed, no sooner was an operation decided on for me than my son had to have two, one following the other. I had always had a dread of hospitals, especially of operations, and waiting for a bed was not easy. However, although because of physical illness I was no longer able to practise moving, I did practise Dr Weekes's teaching to help me through the waiting period. I also practised it in hospital. Those experiences I dreaded most – for example, the pre-operative ritual – lost much of their dreaded value when once I faced and accepted them. Looking back now, I am glad of the experience. I no longer fear hospital so much.

'But I wasn't going to be let off so easily. I had post-operative complications and the journey home from hospital showed me how sensitized I had become. Starting all over again while I felt so weak and sensitized seemed too much. I though I was at the bottom of the ladder and couldn't imagine how I had ever managed to do what I had been doing before entering hospital. I felt so exhausted I didn't even want to recover again. That was that. Period.

'I was making the mistake of being, to quote Dr Weekes, duped by my thinking. I was duped into thinking recovery from this physical illness depended entirely on my effort, when I felt incapable of making effort. Never having had an operation before, I did not know how much physical setback was to be expected, although my surgeon had warned me of some of it. Having come through, I will never again be bluffed by the feelings that follow physical illness.

'Despite myself, nature began to work. Gradually strength came back. I thought, "If I can come out of this, I'll never be so afraid of setback again." I took heart and decided to stop kicking against fate.'

The Old Urge Returned

'Gradually as I felt stronger, the old urge to try once more returned, How much had I lost? The return was gradual. At one stage I hardly dared venture out alone. And just when I was picking up I had an attack of such violent giddiness I was nearly thrown to the floor. This was all I needed to finish me off. Small wonder I hesitated to start again, because my cure lies in being able to drive my car alone. Driving in heavy London traffic is sensitizing in itself without the added fear of having another vertigo attack. However, I was reassured when a specialist told me nothing organic was wrong and that it was most unlikely I would have another attack.

'Also, Dr Weekes explained that unless I tried again I would be left straddling two worlds – the world of agoraphobia and the world of recovery I had glimpsed so well. She was right. That glimpse was my undoing. I just had to go on.

'Of course, I panicked. Noise; traffic; all seemed so much worse than before. But I understood this was to be expected in my condition and I stopped watching my reactions so closely. I even had the sense to stop comparing what I could do now with what I could do in January – three months earlier.

'Gradually I climbed back to some feeling of confidence, as each achievement reminded me of those earlier efforts. I had not forgotten as much as I thought! Indeed, repeating some of the old experiences, like driving round Hyde Park, proved that the early foundation was there. I was soon to find I was now readier for harder undertakings and that is how I am today.

'I am now trying to work without any props, I used to think, "Well, I can always telephone home and someone will come." But now I go off when no one is home. I made little practices at first. One day, with as little contemplation as possible, I went fifteen miles by car. It was a great moment. Don't envy me too much. It was not easy and three days later I made a complete mess of the same journey. But I have learnt one thing. I cannot stay happy when I fail. I have to go out again and correct my mistakes. As Dr Weekes explains, "Recovery lies in repeated doing until the memory of enough achievement replaces defeatist contemplation."'

Head On Pillow, It All Seems Impossible

'Believe me, I still have my full share of defeatist contemplation, especially at night, when, head on pillow, it all seems impossible. But the next day, somehow, I'm at it again, and once in the car, the doing takes over. I know that for complete recovery, the day must come when the umbilical cord between myself and outside support must be completely cut, and this is what I am working at now.'

Although last summer brought much domestic strain to this woman, she has been able to consolidate the progress she had made with agoraphobia. She can now drive alone to golf, seven miles away, and play all day without needing someone near. She recently drove 200 miles and stayed overnight at a country hotel, after attending her son's school concert at night. She was so delighted she cabled me in Australia from the hotel. Best of all, she can now work away from home, staying a full day on her own.

She also goes to concerts, cinemas and shops with her children and when she remembers agoraphobia on these occasions it is to think how she could not once do these things.

The following letter seems to have been written especially for those of you who are determined to come out of your illness by your own effort:

'Today's newspaper carried an article on phobias and I was forcibly reminded of all the help Dr Weekes's journals have brought to me. I simply must write and say that my agoraphobia is almost a thing of the past. Even the trembling attacks that replaced it are no longer important.

'As I strolled through the big stores yesterday, looking at the midi-line, I became aware of what I was doing and of how much I had improved. For one bitter-sweet moment, I thought of all those wasted years when I was trapped. But there must be no looking back, except in gratitude.

'I feel Dr Weekes's method has the same objective as the drug relaxation method, which, although perhaps quicker, would not give the same basic understanding and permanent confidence as did her explanation and encouragement. The drug method is like going out and buying a bunch of flowers. Dr Weeke's method means getting the seeds and growing them yourself – much more rewarding.'

I hope you will all persevere until the prize is yours. If you have the help of an understanding doctor, so much the better. If you have not, I assure you, however much you may have failed in the past, you can still do it on your own. This teaching is not only a cure for nervous illness, it is a way of life – that too was written by a reader of these journals.

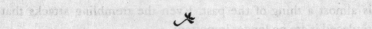

Coming Through Setback

Since I have often mentioned setback in this book, some of the suggestions made previously must inevitably be repeated in what I am now about to say. However, coming through setback is such an important part of recovery that it merits this closing chapter to itself, with any necessary repetition.

IN A GOOD PERIOD THEY GATHER HOPE

Some people on hearing a satisfactory explanation of their illness lose fear of it and recover remarkably quickly. Others may frequently find themselves in a setback. Most nervously ill people are surprised to hear they can make as much progress towards recovery in a setback as in a good spell. In a good period they gather hope and feel the healing effect of peace, but often at the back of their mind lurks the thought that their illness may recur, and of course any remaining sensitization, helped by memory, will certainly do its best to see that 'it' returns from time to time.

THE VERY SIGHT SPELLS WEARINESS

Memory is ready to waylay the nervously ill person at every turn in the road. The sufferer has seen those houses, those streets, those shops, so often, the very sight spells weariness, illness. Each upsetting sensation that memory recalls may awaken such suffering that its victim can easily mistake memory for reality and think he he has slipped to the bottom of the ladder once more. The contrast between the hope and peace experienced in a good spell and the suffering felt in a setback highlights the suffering and makes it seem more unendurable than ever.

This contrast makes the early setbacks seem especially severe and brings deep disappointment. It seems to the sufferer that whenever he tries to go forward, some 'thing' is always ready to drag him back. He had thought that as he recovered, setbacks, if they occurred, would be less and less severe, occur less frequently. And so they may. But the worst setback of all can come just before complete recovery. The nearness of recovery make a setback at this time especially frustrating. And yet, however severe setback may be, if it is coped with the right way, it does not retard ultimate recovery. Try to remember this.

YOU NEED NOT BE WAYLAID BY MEMORY

You should understand the tricks memory and habit can play so that you are not too discouraged by setback, however long it may last or whenever it may come. You should learn to appreciate the difference between memory and reality and know that when memory recalls past suffering and reawakens old tensions, apprehensions, *it is still only memory*, and you need not be waylaid by memory, however painful and convincing it may seem.

Let memory recall as much as it may; but do not let this deceive you into thinking you have slipped into illness again, although for a while you may feel the symptoms as acutely as ever.

GRANDMA'S SCONES

When I was young, Grandma often had a batch of hot scones waiting for me after school. When I smell hot scones now, Grandma immediately comes to mind. I do not think, 'Hot scones! What do they remind me of? Ah, yes! Grandma!' I just automatically think of her.

Setback is like Grandma's scones. Even when you have recovered, if something suddenly recalls your illness you may feel the shadow of past suffering as quickly as I remember those scones. When this happens, if you think, 'Only Grandma's scones!' you will help the shadow of the shadow to pass.

It is the unaccountable suddenness of setback that causes shock, so that the sufferer seems temporarily at least to lose the power to reason with it and to help himself. A woman wrote, 'I have done well with desensitizing myself. I have a return of panic only about once a month now. It is strange that the further apart the spells come, the less I know how to handle them quickly. They come with a greater shock after a long peaceful period and I'm so out of practice that for a while I forget your advice.'

'MY EMOTIONS ARE WIBBLY-WOBBLY WITH THE SHOCK'

Another woman said, 'When a setback strikes, it is sometimes quite a while before I can practise what you have taught me.

The setback seems so engulfing at first. It's difficult to make my attitude positive quickly enough. My emotions are so wibbly-wobbly with the shock of setback, the encouragement I try to give myself doesn't get beyond words. It doesn't register any feeling of belief or bring any relief. I walk round all day giving myself words, words. It takes quite a while before I can feel in charge of the situation again. But this is gradually getting better, as I have more practice. I feel a little more confident each time I find my way out of a setback and I'm beginning to remember the way out more readily.'

UPSETTING SYMPTOMS RETURN SO QUICKLY

One of the most shocking aspects can be the surprisingly quick return of *all* the upsetting symptoms. The sufferer is tempted to think the number of returning symptoms is a measure of the severity of the setback. It is not. If you think of your cousin John, the chances are you will also think of others in the family. This is no more than a chain of related memories. All the symptoms of setback are the symptoms of stress and anxiety, so that their quick reappearance in full – as a family, as it were – simply means you are very anxious again.

Just as the conductor of an orchestra can stop all instruments with one rap of his baton, so you can calm all symptoms with one treatment, acceptance. You do not need a special lotion for your sweating hands; a special tablet for giddiness, another for agitation. A mild tranquillizer *and acceptance* work on them all. So do not watch each symptom anxiously.

REACTIONS WITHOUT SO MUCH FEAR

As understanding and acceptance heal sensitization, feeling will not follow thought so swiftly, intensely, and you will be able to reason less emotionally with your feelings, even less emotionally with panic. Confidence comes from experience and some of your best experience lies in coming through setback; because, as I said earlier, each setback gives yet another opportunity to practise, until you make my teaching part of yourself, make it so inbuilt that your reactions in any future disturbing situation will not be the old frightening flashback reactions, but will gradually be the right ones – reactions without so much shock, fear. You will know the way out of setback so well, you will no longer fear the way in.

'MUST I ALWAYS HAVE SETBACKS?'

This answers the question so often asked, 'Must I always have setbacks?' Setbacks gradually fade from the scene when you no longer fear them. You are completely cured when you no longer fear setback, because when you are unafraid of them they lose their meaning. They become only memory of how you once suffered. Indeed, when you have learnt to cope with a setback, it serves to highlight the progress you have made, and you can then look back on your illness with a sense of gratitude for having had the experience. Oh, yes, this day will come. But this takes time. You must not count each day spent in a setback. You must not think, 'Oh, my goodness! This one's lasted longer than any of the others! *This* will never go!'

If a setback is especially long, you will find it is because you are waiting too impatiently for it to go; you are withdrawing in fear; or are impatiently trying to break your way through it, fight it; have become hopeless about recovering. *You must give as much time to coming through each setback as it demands.* Do not try to force a way through setback, testing yourself each night, each morning, to see if you are feeling any better. Try not to watch yourself too anxiously. This, I know, is not easy, but you can't step out of setback like stepping out of a garment. Let setback have its head. It will certainly take it anyhow, so you may as well give in gracefully and float along with it.

Understand that the more you worry about being in a setback, the more you resensitize yourself and the longer setback will last. I understand how tired you may be of continually trying to get yourself 'up off the floor'. But the more you can do it without too much frustration, the sooner you will find peace.

WELL ONE DAY; ILL THE NEXT

I am often asked why a nervously ill person can feel so well one day and then, for no apparent reason, so ill the next. For example, why an agoraphobic person can travel into town without fear one day, and yet the next day feel the old fears as acutely as ever. Strangely enough, as I stressed in Chapter 3, it is because yesterday's journey was so successful that the nervous person is vulnerable to defeat today. The memory of yesterday's success may make him over-anxious to be just as successful again. So he may start the journey apprehensively, therefore slightly more sensitized than he was yesterday, and it may take only some minor incident on the way into town to bring panic immediately. When this happens, he is convinced this journey will be a failure. So he despairs, and such acute emotion as despair sensitizes still further and makes him more vulnerable to the thought of failure. He is making the mistake of testing himself.

Remember, practise; never test. Do not set an examination for yourself to see if you can travel without panic. If you have panic after panic, and yet try to take each the right way, as far as future recovery is concerned, *the journey made with panic is just as successful as the journey made without it*. Also, if you test yourself, failure brings a sense of defeat; whereas with practice, failure means only that you can practise again. Can you see the difference between testing and practising? The very thought of testing brings tension; whereas the thought of practising holds no urgent demand.

Also, doing the unusual, although it may be no more than boarding a bus, may seem very unreal. So that, in the beginning, even when successful, there may be no feeling of achievement, only a feeling of strangeness. Indeed, one's illness can seem more real than the early stages of recovery, and the journey into town – or any other undertaking – may have to be made successfully many times before it is accompanied by any sense of real achievement. Achievement must be consolidated before you can feel firm ground from which to face the future.

As I said earlier, when you understand the value of repeated achievement, then achievement may become such an urgency that you may be afraid to let a day pass without practising for fear you will lose what you have already gained. You will never lose what you have gained once you practise the right way.

If physical illness brings a halt to your efforts, do not let postponements become a permanent avoidance.

THE ALARMING RETURN OF PANIC

When I review the difficulties of recovery, I would say the most alarming of all is the return of panic weeks, even years, after recovery. In my experience, this unexpected reappearance of panic causes more concern than any other aspect of nervous illness. It shocks, frightens, and it *reminds*. That is why it is so shocking. It reminds one of so much one would rather forget forever; of so much one hoped one had forgotten forever.

The fear immediately added, together with the physical disturbance caused by panic, resensitizes slightly and helps bring back some of the old, perhaps almost forgotten, nervous sensations, so that the unwary sufferer may be bluffed into thinking 'it' has returned, or will return if he doesn't look out.

One woman, after being well for a year, had a return of panic while shopping. She immediately dashed out of the shop and avoided it for weeks. She had once more retreated from fear, in fear.

Never do this. Never let an unexpected return of panic shock you into running away from it. Halt; go slowly. See the panic through and then go quietly on with whatever you are doing. Let the panic come again and again if it wants to. Do not try to switch it off in fear; do not withdraw blindly from it. Understand that some tension, some strain, may have slightly sensitized you once more; or that memory, stirred by some sight, sound, thought, smell, may have flashed the old feeling. Any of us at times may become slightly sensitized by strain, so that we feel on edge, apprehensive. If this happens to one who has felt panic intensely in the past, his apprehension can quickly change to panic, because the way to panic in him is so well worn. One could almost say his panic-mechanism is well oiled, ready.

If you can accept that for a long time to come you may have a strong flash of panic from time to time, and if you can realize this means no more than that you are slightly sensitized for the moment, or that memory has stirred the embers of your illness, and if you can see this panic through for what it is – only a physical feeling without real significance – then you are truly recovered despite occasional bouts of recurring panic.

I remind you again that recovery from panic lies on the other side of panic, whenever it may come. Always see it through and go on with the job in hand. Never run home in fear. Never begin avoiding again.

So:

* Accept everything about your illness.
* Do not waste energy trying to analyse every strange happening.
* Do not be dismayed by setback; nor bluffed by memory.
* Do not despair when achievement seems unreal; practise, never test.
* Do not be overawed by defeatist contemplation.
* Do not be dismayed if you feel nervier than ever when you first begin the journey to recovery.
* Do not be discouraged by physical illness.
* Above all, do not be shocked by return of panic, or any strange flash-experience.

You may think there is so much to remember, so much to do. There isn't, you know. It is all in one word – accept. Once you have the understanding this book brings, it will not matter if you forget the rest, as long as you remember that one little word *accept*. Good luck.

*

Index

DR CLAIRE WEEKES SPEAKS

Dr Weekes gives further help on audio cassettes/CDs and a video/DVD for sufferers from 'nerves'.

The audio cassettes are called:

Hope and Help for Your Nerves
Moving to Freedom, Going on Holiday
Good Night, Good Morning
Nervous Fatigue

The video is called:

Peace from Nervous Suffering

The audio cassettes/CDs (except *Hope and Help for Your Nerves*) are available to the United Kingdom, Ireland and Europe from:

Pacific Recordings
32 Woodside Drive
BINGLEY
West Yorkshire
BD16 1RF
ENGLAND

Tel: +44 (0) 1274 564443

The video/DVD is available to the United Kingdom, Ireland and Europe from:

Pacific Recordings
32 Woodside Drive
BINGLEY
West Yorkshire
BD16 1RF
ENGLAND

Tel: +44 (0) 1274 564443

Rest of the world:

Claire Weekes Publications Pty
Ltd
PO Box 377
Woden ACT 2606
AUSTRALIA

Rest of the world:

Claire Weekes Publications Pty
Ltd
PO Box 377
Woden ACT 2606
AUSTRALIA

Hope and Help for Your Nerves
Available from bookshops or
HarperThorsons Mail Order
Tel: 0870 900 2050